THE VISIONARY PATH

TRANSFORMING STRESS INTO PURPOSE

Nine Steps to a Happy Brain

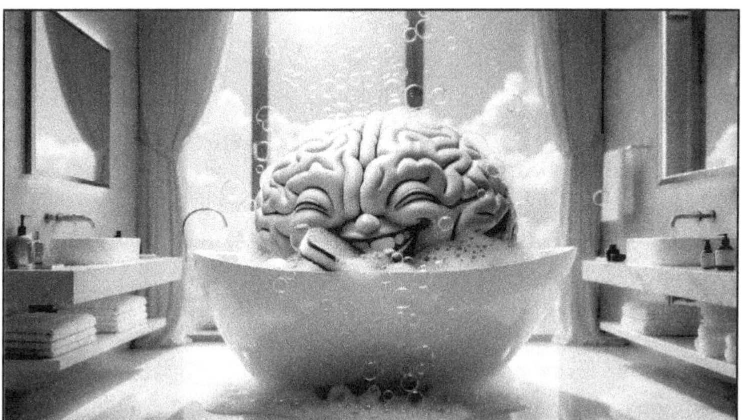

MARIA IAN

SUN CAVE PRODUCTIONS

ISBN Paperback: 979-8-9918862-7-7.

ISBN Ebook: 979-8-9918862-6-0

DEDICATION

To P, who wanted to read my book.

ACKNOWLEDGEMENTS

The author would like to thank the survivors, whether living or dead. Their motivation and unceasing striving served as inspiration for this book.

CONTENTS

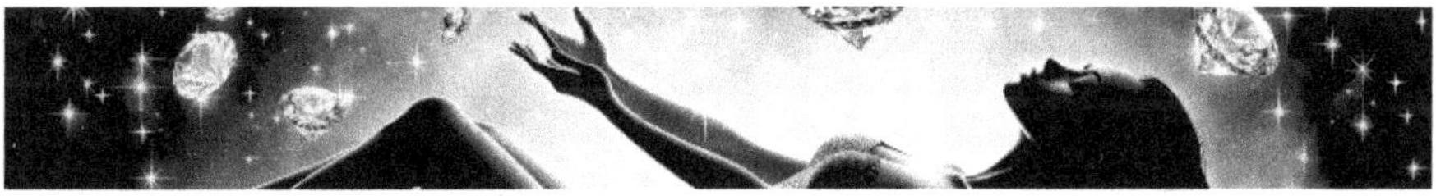

Ignite Your Spirit! Tune Into my VoiceAmerica Media Podcast "The Visionary Path: Transforming Stress Into Purpose. Nine Steps to a Happy Brain" for 13 hours of Electrifying Wisdom, Transformative Insights, And Cosmic Energy

https://caveofthesun.com/podcast-visionary-path-1

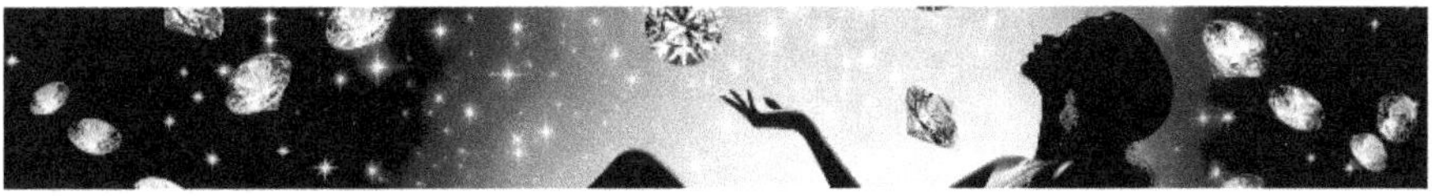

WHAT IS A VISIONARY?

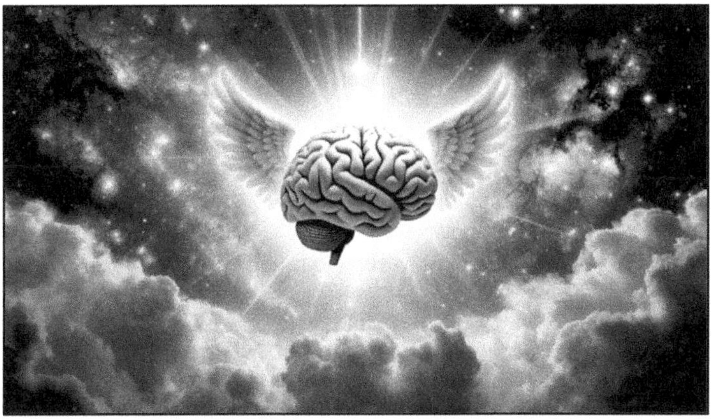

You picked up this book because you are a visionary. You are a soul who dances on the precipice of possibility, a dream-weaver who gazes beyond the veil of the present, an architect of the future, a person who wants to make dreams into tangible realities. Or at least you know you can do all of these things. You know it is within you to make the ordinary an extraordinary experience. You are a doer who wants to illuminate the way to creativity and innovation. You have clarity of mind amidst the chaos.

But at the same time, you are a realist. You know that stress, fear, and anxiety can get in the way. You feel you are on the brink of a great accomplishment, but it's wiser to be cautious, so you pull back. You get nervous when you want to step up for the next great idea; it may not come out right after all. You prepared thoroughly, but the time may not be ripe. Deep down, you think you really should take some rest. You mustn't incur any losses.

That's right – problems are heaping up. Now it's crystal clear to you, why you couldn't take that visionary step. There is so much that still needs to be done. How could you have been so foolish? You wasted your time on a silly dream. You must look at it with wisdom. Things always fall into place, eventually. You shouldn't stress, until then. If you were perfectly honest with yourself, that is the state you are in, right now: You are stressed, very much so.

But you never give up. You burn to transform your reality with focus and purpose. You want to silence your monkey mind. You dream of breaking free from the constant noise that holds you back. You see yourself standing at the edge of your potential, where emotional intelligence transforms into crystal-clear direction. What if I told you extraordinary seeds lie in this chaos of your mind? Can you maintain momentum and stay flexible in the face of this uncertainty?

Within you lies the rare ability to pierce through the static of everyday noise and extract the pure signal of opportunity. It's a journey of awakening, not a question of your capability. It's called unleashing your natural but dormant gifts so you can take the risk purposefully and turn your vision into a living truth. This book will lay the stepping stones so you can face the stormy sea confidently, hold on to your values, and come out at the other end intact, transformed, and greatly improved.

Let's begin by looking into details at what a visionary is. I bet you have known at least one person who left an indelible imprint on your life when you least expected it, or you noticed it only much later. A visionary doesn't have to be famous. While many famous people are visionaries, this quality may not always thrive in the limelight. Being a visionary certainly does not require fame; the qualities of a visionary can be found in anyone, whether that would be someone in your family, among your friends and acquaintances, or a colleague at work. Not everyone, however, can use and make real the qualities of a visionary – calm, focus, mental clarity, far-sightedness, creativity, a knack for finding the way out of adversity. Yet each one of us has these abilities. Sometimes you can feel surrounded by these little sparks.

How many times have you wished you could quiet your monkey mind? Complete that vital project? Start on the new route you have set your eyes on for so long? Push just a little bit more beyond that boundary? Not let fear and stress intimidate you just then when it counts? Navigate the turbulent waters of your life as the captain at *your* helm? You put yourself in those situations and asked those questions precisely because you are a visionary.

If there is one quality that trumps all the others in the sense that it embodies them all, then thriving in adversity tops the list. You've had that churning feeling of an archer the nanosecond before he shoots the arrow. I bet you've had that feeling not once but many times. Most times, you thought it was anxiety; it may have caused you stress and aggravation, and you wished you could have just let it pass on its way. I want to tell you an anecdote that you will much appreciate

A champion challenged a Zen Master who was renowned for his skill as an archer. The young man demonstrated remarkable technical proficiency when he hit a distant bull's eye on his first try. "There," he said to the old man, "see if you can match that!"

Undisturbed, the old man did not draw his bow but motioned to the young man to follow him up a mountain. They reached a deep chasm, where the old man stepped out onto the middle of an unsteady and perilous bridge, picked a faraway tree on the opposite bank as a target, drew his bow, and fired a clean hit. "Now it is your turn," he said as he stepped back onto the safe ground.

Staring with terror into the seemingly bottomless, beckoning abyss, the young man faltered at stepping out onto the log; much less was he able to shoot at the target.

"You have much skill with your bow," the master said, sensing his challenger's predicament, "but you have little skill with the mind that lets loose the shot."

That's a pity because what you, the champion, experience when you want to set foot onto the bridge is the essence, the precious quality of being human. You may be interested to know that what sets the quality of being a visionary apart from all your other attributes is that unless you properly train this quality, it will be useless. It can lie dormant for long periods. You experience terror when you are ready to take the right step.

You may have felt that something inside you has gone missing in the basement, in the ditches, by the roadside, in your subconscious. You may have tried to implement your precious quality of a visionary and concluded it did you more harm than good. So you may have accustomed yourself to avoiding that. Many people who are used to suffering, being miserable, and beating themselves up do not know how to hone their visionary qualities.

We don't need training to eat, sleep, leave the cave, and migrate; in modern times, we still do the same and act out various impulses daily. These many mechanical but labor-intensive, focused routines of our workdays can govern our daily lives. Those activities already take up so much effort; with all the work we put into our daily living, we must do it right after all.

Intriguingly, the prospect of piercing through the present to see the future, creating new worlds, and living our dreams to many of us can appear more straightforward and faster to achieve than the daily grind in the woods. How quickly, after all, can a good book or movie move you? How fast are you transported into realms of imagination, to the what-should-have-been? It can be perfectly justified for you to want to be somewhere other than where you are.

The opposite is true: You are seriously misdirecting your attention. This book will guide you to focus on your visionary qualities so that when you interact with the mundane, you will gain instead of deplete your strength. By making your visionary quality into the real you, you will be more yourself when you apply and use that quality. The daily grind may slowly start to look very different as well.

I wrote this book as a tribute to the visionaries in my life. When I started this book, I planned to write about the highly interesting experiences of survivors of war zones, whether of combat zones or of the ruthless torture environments that characterize some forms of imprisonment. But I quickly realized the guiding thread uniting these experiences was the peculiar mental and emotional calm of persons who had lived through horrific events.

Many decades ago, when I first encountered such persons as a child, that highly special dimension to their being initially led me to disbelieve them strongly. I was led to believe they are not of this world; it would be best to ignore them. I made a grave mistake; such people can teach priceless life lessons. The first experiences were with both of my parents and my grandmother, who were survivors of World War II labor camps, many forced deportations, and combat zones.

I was about five years old and was taken to the emergency room with a severe lymph knot infection that required an operation. I was afraid of telling my father I was so sick; I thought he would be very angry that I had been careless with my health. But to the complete contrary, he drove me to the hospital as if on thin air on angel's wings. I was utterly baffled as to why he would be so calm and so deeply silently attentive towards me instead of worried and upset.

My experiences with my grandmother were not only otherworldly but uncanny. She lost her family to the Bolshevik Revolution and, as a child, had to migrate on foot from Uzbekistan to Eastern Europe. Not to speak that, as a child, she had to walk long distances, wear insufficient clothing in the snow, go to school, and sleep in trees to avoid dangerous individuals. I thought it was sadistic or eminently disrespectful when she recounted the many deaths and disappearances of loved ones she had witnessed in a tone that evidenced spiritual satisfaction and even emotional well-being.

But I was severely wrong in feeling judgmental. It would take decades for me to notice that her capacity for storytelling encompassed observations about relations between Russia and Ukraine that, a century later, have slowly shown themselves to be true. After an eminently stressful life, she died a week short of her one-hundredth birthday.

More recently, I walked into what was to be a meeting with a client of my law firm who, as a combatant, had lived through some of the most horrific wars in the Middle East. I expected a nasty, mean-looking person, someone used to being armed to the teeth. Yet, the person I saw was disarmingly friendly and appeared professionally meditative, calm, and joyful. That caused me to almost stumble backward out of the room; at least the person evoked too much respect for me to enter it. There are many other examples. Interestingly, they are not restricted to any age or gender.

So, you will ask yourself, "Do I have to go to and survive a war zone so I can feel timeless, achieve a heightened sense of well-being, be calm, clear, and focused, and leave my mark on the world?" The good news is you don't have to. There is even better news: You don't have to because, by being human, each of us is both a war zone and a visionary inside of him or herself. Each of us inside has all of the unknown threats, anxieties, fears, and stressors required; they are as old as humankind. You don't have to go anywhere to change your existence in the trenches into the best version of yourself and to transform the trenches into the life of your dreams. All it takes is your sincere willingness to engage with some pervasive factors of cognitive neuroscience – and with the eternal human truths behind them.

This book contains language that can strike you as a little on the technical, medical side at times, but you must remember: It is all for your benefit. You are not just a ball of flesh and bones, and indeed, you aren't bothered if you are referred to as made of two arms, two legs, a trunk, and a head. You aren't worried because any such reference appears obviously true to you. It's the medical language, on the other hand, that seems outlandish. But it is the reverse: The true you is the visionary this language will reveal. It is this true you that transforms the reality of flesh and bones. So you shouldn't object to being referred to as made of the stuff that cognitive neuroscience talks about. The use of medical language is kept to a minimum in this book. When you encounter it, it is a tribute to who you are as a human.

A Note on How to Make Best Use of The Exercises in This Book

The exercises in this book are an invitation to self-exploration. You are invited to reflect and write about yourself. You should not approach this as multiple choice or short answers responses. The exercises are meant as assistance to you to succinctly capture your perceptions, thoughts, and emotions so you can learn about and make better use of your authentic self.

A lot of writing is not required, but you should commit to set aside short periods of undisturbed, quiet time. Humans are made for narration; we could not have survived as a species without storytelling. There is no better way to start than with yourself.

What Does Mindfulness Mean?

You have come to know mindfulness as the practice of intentionally focusing attention on the present moment, observing thoughts, feelings, and sensations without judgment. You cultivate awareness of your internal and external experiences, promoting a state of openness, curiosity, and acceptance.[1] The term "mindfulness" comes up often in this book. The experience is assisted by the means of meditation.

---

[1] Mindfulness, https://www.apa.org/topics/mindfulness

You will now learn that it is so much more. Mindfulness engages executive functions, enhancing attention control, emotional regulation, and metacognitive awareness.[2] Mindfulness practice reconfigures brain networks, particularly the executive control, default mode, and salience networks, improving cognitive flexibility and information processing.[3] This perspective emphasizes a skill that strengthens neural pathways, promoting adaptive responses to stress in addition to enhancing overall cognitive performance.

You will notice this as you read this book. So look at the term "mindfulness" in the context in which you encounter it, as a term of activity, empowerment and confidence.

---

[2] Sars D (2022) PE augmented mindfulness: A neurocognitive framework for research and future healthcare. Front. Hum. Neurosci. 16:899988. doi: 10.3389/fnhum.2022.899988

[3] Yue WL, Ng KK, Koh AJ, Perini F, Doshi K, Zhou JH, Lim J. Mindfulness-based therapy improves brain functional network reconfiguration efficiency. Transl Psychiatry. 2023 Nov 11;13(1):345. doi: 10.1038/s41398-023-02642-9. PMID: 37951943; PMCID: PMC10640625.

YOU HAVE WHAT IT TAKES

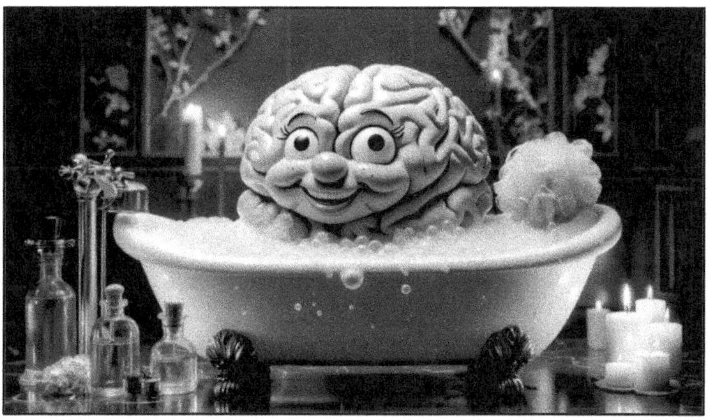

Our journey starts with the basics. Do you have a burning interest in self-help? Most likely, you have heard of the survival mind, and most likely, that idea left you deeply dissatisfied. The survival mind is that part of us that wants to keep us safe, as it is crucial for our evolution as a species. The survival mind resists the unfamiliar and causes you much fear and stress. You would much rather have that other, undeniable power of a visionary; you know nature made you excel and seek new horizons. So, you are torn between the two and troubled in deciding which works best. You could say nature has built you up for failure. But that's the generalization.

You are most likely now asking yourself why you experience fear and stress then when you want to keep yourself safe. "Shouldn't I just excel, chart new paths for myself, and leave the old behind?" you ask. But that won't work, as you quickly find out. For one, you realize you may not need all that extra effort and exertion; safety, after all, is appealing and cozy for you. Who cares about the stress? It will certainly soon pass and leave your nice, warm corner. It is that horrible stress and fear you must avoid at all costs. It creeps up on you each time you want to peek into what's next. Why venture beyond if that is the price to be paid? It is much better to listen to your body and mind wisely and stay where you are!

We humans are needy creatures; even if, to keep ourselves safe, we were to hide underneath a blanket inside the closet, it is precisely the blanket and the darkness of the closet that we crave. The situation gives us a sense of control, which we experience as rewarding, like comfort food. And that is only one-half of the picture. To be hardwired for failure, pulled into the closet while we want to excel, also means to be hardwired for the fear and stress that come with this failure, which in turn means that craving conditions of fear and stress can't be the end goal of any human life. We humans are so made that we just always crave – something.

Here comes cognitive neuroscience to tell you that what you thought was right is, in fact, very wrong. Individuals with higher psychological resilience show lower activity in the area of their brains, which modulates emotional responses and reward processing. This reduced activity is not a sign of diminished function but rather an indication of enhanced control of quick emotional reactions. It allows resilient individuals to maintain a clear head and make sound decisions even when faced with life-threatening situations.[4] Resilience plays a crucial role in the calm and visionary mindset.

---

[4] Kong F, Ma X, You X, Xiang Y. The resilient brain: psychological resilience mediates the effect of amplitude of low-frequency fluctuations in orbitofrontal cortex on subjective well-being in young healthy

"What?" you say. "You meant to tell me that when I felt so strong in my safety, I was buried in a closet and very weak instead?" Yes, that's precisely what I just said.

One of the most striking characteristics of resilient individuals is their ability to remain calm under extreme pressure. When exposed to threatening stimuli, they often display altered activity in the amygdala and insula.[5] These brain regions are typically associated with fear and anxiety responses. In resilient individuals, however, these areas show more regulated activity. This neural calm translates into behavioral and cognitive benefits. Veterans of wars and other survivors often report an ability to "slow down time" during critical moments, allowing for clearer thinking and more precise actions. This phenomenon is likely related to enhanced activity in the prefrontal cortex, which is responsible for executive functions such as decision-making and, importantly, impulse control.

Perhaps even more remarkable than the ability to stay calm is the capacity for visionary and creative thinking some individuals develop in high-risk environments. This seemingly paradoxical response to danger is rooted in the brain's plasticity and ability to form new neural connections in response to extreme experiences. Exposure to severe stress can enhance connectivity between different brain regions, particularly those involved in problem-solving and abstract thinking.[6]

This increased neural cross-talk may explain why some war zone survivors report moments of profound insight or innovative solutions to life-threatening problems. The experience of surviving extreme danger often leads to a shift in perspective. Many survivors report a heightened

---

adults. Soc Cogn Affect Neurosci. 2018 Sep 4;13(7):755-763. doi: 10.1093/scan/nsy045. PMID: 29939335; PMCID: PMC6121151.

[5] Palamarchuk IS and Vaillancourt T (2021) Mental Resilience and Coping With Stress: A Comprehensive, Multi-level Model of Cognitive Processing, Decision Making, and Behavior. Front. Behav. Neurosci. 15:719674. doi: 10.3389/fnbeh.2021.719674

[6] Learning to stay calm in life-threatening situations, January 16, 2024, https://www.maastrichtuniversity.nl/news/learning-stay-calm-life-threatening-situations

sense of purpose and a clearer vision of what truly matters in life. This psychological transformation is likely underpinned by changes in the default mode network, a set of brain regions involved in self-reflection and long-term planning.[7]

So what's missing in the picture of the needy you craving the safety of the closet? We'll start at the most elementary, where we encounter what you – and everyone else - decided to do at that moment. Keep this before your eyes: Your brain can adapt to extreme stress and develop visionary qualities. You can choose to find excuses, fall back, and ultimately die, or you can choose to adapt. Choosing to die is not an excuse for not choosing to adapt. A human being never truly or eternally dies. The energy that supports you changes its form on its continuum of eternity. Something else is always at work. It is what you make of the energy that you are that matters. Do you still want to choose to die? All you will have accomplished is many problems, blockages, barriers, and distortions in the world you have left behind. While the problem that is you just continues on and on, on its eternal path.

At its most elementary level, human life is replete with the choices we face at every moment of our lives in our ever-changing environments. From the mundane decisions of what to eat for breakfast to life-altering career moves, your ability to choose shapes your experiences and defines your reality. Making a choice recruits neural circuitry in your brain that is involved in reward and motivation processing.[8] These are also involved in your craving for safety. "So everything is fine, after all, and I don't have to do much?" you will ask.

---

[7] Kong F, Ma X, You X, Xiang Y. The resilient brain: psychological resilience mediates the effect of amplitude of low-frequency fluctuations in orbitofrontal cortex on subjective well-being in young healthy adults. Soc Cogn Affect Neurosci. 2018 Sep 4;13(7):755-763. doi: 10.1093/scan/nsy045. PMID: 29939335; PMCID: PMC6121151.

[8] Leotti LA, Iyengar SS, Ochsner KN. Born to choose: the origins and value of the need for control. Trends Cogn Sci. 2010 Oct;14(10):457-63. doi: 10.1016/j.tics.2010.08.001. PMID: 20817592; PMCID: PMC2944661.

Nothing could be further from the truth. There is a being, a YOU, that does the craving. When you make a choice, your brain also integrates information about value and personal relevance. That brain region is more active when making self-relevant choices than simple perceptual discriminations. Meanwhile, a part of the brain's reward system shows increased activity when options are available, suggesting that choosing may be inherently rewarding.

So, humans are wired to experience our choices as both relevant to ourselves and inherently rewarding. Now, think for a second about what you are telling yourself when you choose safety in the closet. You get a kick out of telling yourself that you are no good. I am not hurting your feelings by revealing this to you; you already are sufficiently hurting yourself. By choosing the closet, you reward yourself with an awful place.

Having the power of choice has been shown to create an illusion of control. There is a reason why it doesn't bother you to be in a bad place; the closet allows you to manage the fear that would otherwise inundate you from all sides. However, we humans tend to overestimate our control over outcomes. The illusion of control may serve a protective function. We would just not opt for certain things as they could undermine our experience of control. There are certain cases, of course, where that can be good, such as avoiding maladaptive cognitive and affective responses.

When provided with choices, the default assumption of control is deeply ingrained in our human cognition. This tendency is observed across various populations, including preschool-aged children and even non-human primates. The persistence of this effect, even in amnesic patients who can't explicitly remember making a choice, suggests that it operates at a fundamental, implicit level of cognition.[9] Making choices daily in our ever-changing environments is a necessity that allows us to experience control over these environments in a self-relevant and rewarding way.

---

[9] Id.

The ability to make choices is intimately linked with emotional regulation and, interestingly, also with long-term planning. You imagine future outcomes and guide your decisions accordingly. This gradual ramping up of neural activity during decision-making provides flexibility in your responses, allowing you to modulate your choices based on the accumulated evidence. And that's a good thing since, at least in theory, you are never truly lost. A person who perceives their state of failure as genuinely rewarding can still have the flexibility to adapt to the horizon beyond. It's just that because of various mistaken factors, the person may choose not to do so.

Any situation you find yourself in is, to a large extent, a product of your past choices. And the past does not have to be a distant place. It can be the last second when you decide to fall back into darkness; that second can turn pervasive and permanent. Have you ever had an experience as simple as wanting to get up from your desk but something keeping you back? Did an unfavorable sentiment then develop that subsequently, somehow, pulled in its wake other, more extraordinary unfavorable sentiments?

It is important to emphasize that the beliefs you choose to hold, consciously or unconsciously, shape your experiences and the opportunities you perceive. You are created for a flexible process. Your brain constantly predicts and simulates potential futures based on your past experiences and current beliefs.[10] Different brain regions are implicated in representing various aspects of decision values,[11] such as the primary value difference based on likely outcomes and the secondary value differences associated with less likely scenarios. This dual

[10] What's Going on in Our Brains When we Plan? By James Devitt, June 7, 2024, https://www.nyu.edu/about/news-publications/news/2024/june/what-s-going-on-in-our-brains-when-we-plan-.html

[11] Decision-Making with Predictions of Others' Likely and Unlikely Choices in the Human Brain
Ning Ma, Norihiro Harasawa, Kenichi Ueno, Kang Cheng, Hiroyuki Nakahara
Journal of Neuroscience 11 September 2024, 44 (37) e2236232024; **DOI:** 10.1523/JNEUROSCI.2236-23.2024

representation allows for flexible decision-making that accounts for probable and improbable outcomes.

When faced with the worst life throws at you, it's crucial to recognize that your response is a choice. By consciously choosing to adopt a growth mindset and viewing challenges as opportunities for learning, you can reshape your neural circuitry to support more adaptive behaviors.[12] The brain's plasticity allows for the formation of new neural pathways, enabling you to change your habitual responses over time. You don't have to stay in the worst place you perceive as the most rewarding to you until … Correct, not even in that place. You don't have to wait until your present has become unbearably painful to make a change.

You have the neural machinery to support venturing into new territories and breaking out of the old when you choose. And when you make a conscious choice to respond differently to a situation, you strengthen new neural pathways. Importantly, you have the power to explore new options; you don't have to exploit the known rewards.[13] You can harness this power to shape your experiences, overcome challenges, and create your desired life. Instead of viewing yourself as the victim of circumstance, you can see yourself as an active participant in your growth and recovery. This sense of agency is a powerful tool in overcoming adversity and building resilience.

One of the most significant areas where choice plays a role is your emotional responses. You may not always choose your initial emotional reactions, but you have a choice in managing and responding to these emotions.[14] You can develop awareness of your emotional triggers and learn to pause before becoming stressed. This pause allows you to choose

---

[12] Id.

[13] Dennison JB, Sazhin D, Smith DV. Decision neuroscience and neuroeconomics: Recent progress and ongoing challenges. Wiley Interdiscip Rev Cogn Sci. 2022 May;13(3):e1589. doi: 10.1002/wcs.1589. Epub 2022 Feb 8. PMID: 35137549; PMCID: PMC9124684.

[14] Choice, at https://www.cognitivebehavioralcenter.com/choice-

a response that aligns with your values and long-term goals instead of being driven by immediate emotional impulses.

Here are some tips to harness the power of choice in your life:

1. **Regularly examine your core beliefs** and challenge those that you notice limit you.
2. When faced with challenges, **consciously choose a growth-oriented perspective**.
3. **Develop emotional regulation skills** to make more deliberate choices in stressful situations.
4. **Embrace Uncertainty**: Individuals with higher cognitive flexibility tend to exhibit enhanced adaptability and resilience when faced with challenges.[15] Cultivating a tolerance for uncertainty can help you approach new situations with an open mind.
5. **Practice Mindfulness**: Mindfulness is a significant predictor of self-regulation, which is closely linked to cognitive flexibility.[16] Incorporating mindfulness practices into your daily routine can enhance your ability to make conscious choices.
6. **Engage in Novel Experiences**: Exposing yourself to new and diverse situations can strengthen neural pathways associated with cognitive flexibility.[17] This can include learning new skills, exploring different cultures, or engaging in creative pursuits.
7. **Develop Metacognitive Awareness**: Being aware of your thought processes can help you identify and challenge rigid

[15] Nakhostin-Khayyat M, Borjali M, Zeinali M, Fardi D, Montazeri A. The relationship between self-regulation, cognitive flexibility, and resilience among students: a structural equation modeling. BMC Psychol. 2024 Jun 7;12(1):337. doi: 10.1186/s40359-024-01843-1. PMID: 38849898; PMCID: PMC11162044.

[16] Nakhostin-Khayyat M, Borjali M, Zeinali M, Fardi D, Montazeri A. The relationship between self-regulation, cognitive flexibility, and resilience among students: a structural equation modeling. BMC Psychol. 2024 Jun 7;12(1):337. doi: 10.1186/s40359-024-01843-1. PMID: 38849898; PMCID: PMC11162044.

[17] New Research Reveals Close Connection Between Cognitive Flexibility and Neurogenesis, https://news.stonybrook.edu/newsroom/press-release/medical/new-research-reveals-close-connection-between-cognitive-flexibility-and-neurogenesis/

thinking patterns. This metacognitive skill is crucial for adapting to new information and changing circumstances.[18] In our daily lives, we often underestimate the impact of small choices, believing that these minor decisions have little consequence. However, seemingly insignificant choices can profoundly shape your life's trajectory, often in ways you fail to anticipate. Your decision-making process is governed by two distinct cognitive systems: System 1 and System 2.[19] System 1 is fast, intuitive, and emotional, while System 2 is slower, more deliberative, and logical. When making small, everyday choices, we tend to rely heavily on System 1, which can lead to impulsive decisions that may not align with our long-term goals.

Under cognitive load especially, our ability to make reasoned decisions diminishes.[20] This is particularly relevant to small choices, as we often make these decisions while juggling multiple possible outcomes or when stress has depleted our cognitive resources. As a result, we may opt for choices that provide immediate gratification rather than those that benefit us in the long run.

While individual small choices may seem inconsequential, their cumulative effect over time can be substantial. Just as small positive habits can lead to significant improvements, a series of poor choices can gradually steer us off course. Repeated behaviors, even small ones, create neural pathways that reinforce these actions.[21] This means that each small

---

[18] Zühlsdorff K, Dalley JW, Robbins TW, Morein-Zamir S. Cognitive flexibility: neurobehavioral correlates of changing one's mind. Cereb Cortex. 2023 Apr 25;33(9):5436-5446. doi: 10.1093/cercor/bhac431. PMID: 36368894; PMCID: PMC10152092.

[19] Misuraca R, Nixon AE, Miceli S, Di Stefano G and Scaffidi Abbate C (2024) On the advantages and disadvantages of choice: future research directions in choice overload and its moderators. *Front. Psychol.* 15:1290359. doi: 10.3389/fpsyg.2024.1290359

[20] The Effects of Different Cognitive Manipulations on Decision Making, March 27, 2017, https://bpb-us-e2.wpmucdn.com/sites.utdallas.edu/dist/8/1090/files/2022/03/cary_deck_paper.pdf

[21] Savioni, L., Triberti, S., Durosini, I. *et al.* How to make big decisions: A cross-sectional study on the decision making process in life choices. *Curr Psychol* **42**, 15223–15236 (2023). https://doi.org/10.1007/s12144-022-02792-x

choice we make affects our immediate circumstances and shapes our future decision-making patterns.

Not surprisingly, you face uncertainty when faced with incomplete information, outcome variability, or competing choices.[22] [23] Uncertainty is a fundamental aspect of our modern environment and decision-making processes. And the probabilities of potential outcomes are undoubtedly unknown to you when you are underneath your blanket in the closet. The typical response to this ambiguity is anxiety.[24] You are uncertain about the current state of the environment and about the timing of future events, including rewards.[25] You get hyperactive and collect more information, often at a cost,[26] while your actions have increased variability and unsteadiness.[27] You may have encountered the term 'existentialist anxiety' before. Now you know its basics.

Your life in uncertain environments with many small competing choices is prey to poor impulse control. Immediate gratification guides you; that gradually steers you off course. You may underestimate the impact of small choices because of your illusion of control. You tend to believe that, especially since the present is temporary, you can quickly correct our course in the future. That can lead you to be less cautious about your present decisions. Importantly, your belief in your abilities to

---

[22] Topel S, Ma I, Sleutels J, van Steenbergen H, de Bruijn ERA, van Duijvenvoorde ACK. Expecting the unexpected: a review of learning under uncertainty across development. Cogn Affect Behav Neurosci. 2023 Jun;23(3):718-738. doi: 10.3758/s13415-023-01098-0. Epub 2023 May 26. PMID: 37237092; PMCID: PMC10390612.

[23] Levy, I., Schiller, D. Uncertainty in learning and decision-making: Introduction to the special issue. *Cogn Affect Behav Neurosci* **23**, 459–464 (2023). https://doi.org/10.3758/s13415-023-01111-6

[24] Keller, A.M., Taylor, H.A. & Brunyé, T.T. Uncertainty promotes information-seeking actions, but what information?. *Cogn. Research* **5**, 42 (2020). https://doi.org/10.1186/s41235-020-00245-2

[25] Levy, I., Schiller, D. Uncertainty in learning and decision-making: Introduction to the special issue. *Cogn Affect Behav Neurosci* **23**, 459–464 (2023). https://doi.org/10.3758/s13415-023-01111-6

[26] Bahaaeddin Attaallah, Pierre Petitet, Elista Slavkova, Vicky Turner, Youssuf Saleh, Sanjay G Manohar, Masud Husain (2022) Hyperreactivity to uncertainty is a key feature of subjective cognitive impairment eLife 11:e75834
https://doi.org/10.7554/eLife.75834

[27] Keller, A.M., Taylor, H.A. & Brunyé, T.T. Uncertainty promotes information-seeking actions, but what information?. *Cogn. Research* **5**, 42 (2020). https://doi.org/10.1186/s41235-020-00245-2

predict future outcomes is often flawed, a phenomenon known as affective forecasting.[28] You tend to overestimate your future willpower and underestimate the power of habit formation. Have you ever made a choice you feel you could regret but think the choice is necessary, and you can just fix any unwanted results? Our lives can be full of cascades of poor choices that gradually accumulate, pushing us further from our intended path.

Several cognitive biases can influence your small choices:

1. **Present Bias**: You tend to prioritize immediate rewards over future benefits.[29] Small choices feel good in the moment but may not serve your long-term interests.
2. **Confirmation Bias**: You seek information that confirms your existing beliefs.[30] This can prevent you from recognizing the negative impact of your small choices.
3. **Availability Heuristic**: You base your judgments on readily available information.[31] This can cause you to underestimate the long-term consequences of your choices.

Consider these strategies for better decision-making:

1. **Increase Awareness**: Be mindful of the small decisions you make daily. Recognize that each choice contributes to your life's direction, no matter how small.
2. **Engage System 2**: Try to engage your deliberative thinking process for important, small decisions. Take a moment to consider the long-term implications of your choices.

---

[28] Savioni, L., Triberti, S., Durosini, I. *et al.* How to make big decisions: A cross-sectional study on the decision making process in life choices. *Curr Psychol* **42**, 15223–15236 (2023). https://doi.org/10.1007/s12144-022-02792-x

[29] Small Decisions: Using Cognitive Science to Improve Communication with Workers, by Ryan Campbell, https://synergist.aiha.org/202003-small-decisions

[30] Savioni, L., Triberti, S., Durosini, I. *et al.* How to make big decisions: A cross-sectional study on the decision making process in life choices. *Curr Psychol* **42**, 15223–15236 (2023). https://doi.org/10.1007/s12144-022-02792-x

[31] Small Decisions: Using Cognitive Science to Improve Communication with Workers, by Ryan Campbell, https://synergist.aiha.org/202003-small-decisions

3. **Create Positive Habits**: Leverage the compound effect by consciously making small positive choices consistently. Over time, these will accumulate into significant positive outcomes.
4. **Engage in Regular Self-Reflection**: Periodically assess your choices and their alignment with your long-term goals. This can help you identify and correct any deviations early.

Your life in the many scenarios of uncertainty you encounter daily is a life battled by competing choices and governed by immediate and potentially conflicting rewards. You don't have much time to choose. It is a life of illusory control over your circumstances. Such a life looks entirely unlike the existence of the visionary creator you aspire to embrace. In the bias it tends to create for taking the wrong path, this life leads you to break the primary promise you set out with originally on this path called life: The promise you made to yourself to be a visionary creator.

Broken promises and unkept agreements have a profound impact on our decision-making processes.[32] Have you ever been stuck on a project that burns you out with the effort required – after all, you may be about to complete it soon? There is just additional work still needed! Broken promises lead to the formation of large subconscious loops. These mental patterns, operating beneath your conscious awareness, can significantly influence your choices and behaviors in ways you don't fully comprehend. You are unaware of how pervasively you are leading yourself astray.

These loops may manifest as:

- Increased cognitive load and decision fatigue
- Heightened internal conflict during future decision-making processes

[32] *The Four Agreements, A Practical Guide to Personal Freedom,* by Don Miguel Ruiz, Amber-Allen Publishing, Incorporated, 1997.

- Reduced ability to respond effectively to reasons and moral considerations
- Potential development of maladaptive decision-making patterns

The act of breaking a promise is associated with significant cognitive conflict. Individuals who break promises exhibit curved trajectories in their decision-making process, leading to long, extensive, unfinished projects, resulting in burnout and frustration. Individuals who break promises also indicate a higher level of internal conflict than those who keep their promises.[33] This conflict arises from the tension between the desire to act reasonably and the temptation of potential benefits from breaking the agreement. Clearly, quick rewards tempt us over the new options that could be presented if we were to keep our word. Interestingly, those who occasionally break promises experience conflict regardless of any final decision they may make to try to revert to the right path.[34]

Exercises For Making Better Choices When You Are Overwhelmed

1. Mindful Breathing For Cognitive Clarity

Take 3-5 minutes to practice slow, deep breathing before making a decision. Focus on your breath, inhaling for 4 counts and exhaling for 6 counts. Then imagine yourself one year from now and ask yourself how important this decision will seem then.

2. Consequence Mapping For Working Memory and Cognitive Flexibility

On a piece of paper, write down in the left hand column the decision you must make in the form of a question. Add your decision options in columns towards the right. Underneath each option, list potential short-term and long-term consequences.

---

[33] Calluso C, Saulin A, Baumgartner T and Knoch D (2018) Distinct Patterns of Cognitive Conflict Dynamics in Promise Keepers and Promise Breakers. *Front. Psychol.* 9:939. doi: 10.3389/fpsyg.2018.00939

[34] Id.

3. Emotional Labeling to Reduce The Impact of Emotional Reactivity

Before making a decision, identify and label your current emotions. For example, "I feel anxious" or "I feel overwhelmed."

4. Pros and Cons Analysis to Engage Analytical Thinking

On a piece of paper, write down the decision you must make in the form of a question at the top. Underneath, create a simple table with columns for each option. Underneath each option, create an additional table with "Pros" and "Cons." List the advantages and disadvantages.

THE CURSE OF FASCINATION

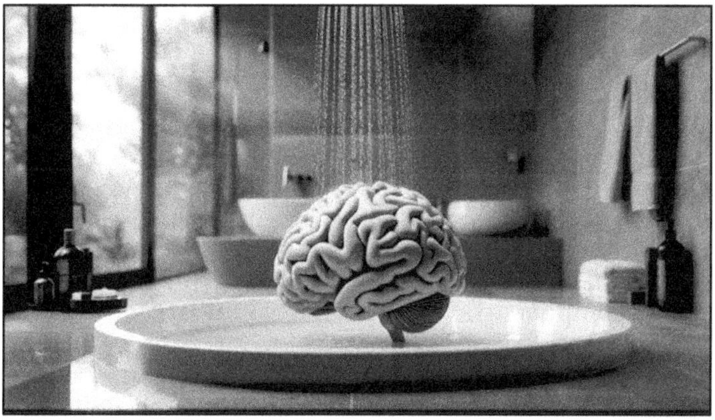

Have you ever felt lost in the enchanted forest? "Oh yes," you will say. "The enchanted forest is, without doubt, the most attractive, appealing place I have ever been to" - but that's not for the reasons you so beautifully imagined! The enchanted forest is located in your subconscious or unconscious mind. It is in the attraction you experience when life entices you to find your way in the world.

You will now be horrified to find out that the enchanted forest is a place of threats, fears, and stress. That's right, you can't escape what landed you in the closet. But you are now about to find out that there is much more! The enchanted forest is the siren that makes your storytelling capacity sing – and you want to be seduced by this siren, right? Then listen up so you can do that the right way!

Invisible, unexpected dangers threaten you there when you feel you have taken refuge. You don't know what hides behind the rustling in the leaves. So beset by anxiety and fear, you follow your impulses for quick rewards that will give you a sense of control over this uncertainty, and who cares if that is illusory? Your rewards are self-relevant in a needy, protective way. The entirety of humanity is with you in this place of doubts; such is the unconscious mind of all of us when stressed and overwhelmed; it goes astray in decision-making. It is very much the ground of a war zone – for the untrained person.

The unconscious mind plays a crucial role in decision-making, more so than previously believed. You have several independent subconscious behavioral guidance systems, including perceptual, evaluative, and motivational components.[35] You perceive, evaluate, and are motivated even then when you are unaware that you are. Your unconscious mind is highly flexible and adaptive, capable of responding to complex situations and influencing your choices and actions in subtle yet powerful ways. Unconscious goal pursuit can produce outcomes.[36] You should not be surprised if your worst nightmare becomes a reality.

Once activated, unconscious goals can guide thoughts and behaviors over extended periods without you consciously intending or monitoring them; that can bear rough weather for you. A tiny but key brain region plays a crucial role in processing uncertainty and is also a significant factor in decisions made in the context of broken promises. The enchanted forest is rife with broken promises: heeding its call can rapidly transform

[35] Bargh JA, Morsella E. The Unconscious Mind. Perspect Psychol Sci. 2008 Jan;3(1):73-9. doi: 10.1111/j.1745-6916.2008.00064.x. PMID: 18584056; PMCID: PMC2440575.
[36] Id.

into the first promise you break, the promise you made to yourself to be a visionary creator!

The same brain region (the lateral habenula) is a major regulator of dopamine. It is linked to mental illnesses such as depression, anxiety, and obsessive-compulsive disorder.[37] It should not surprise you that you can exhibit what can appear to be these conditions when you are astray in the enchanted forest. Fear of uncertainty and the quick rewards your impulses suggest govern you instead of the creativity of new choices. It is an addictive situation; you are rewarded by the illusion of control, after all, so you can always want more.

Meanwhile, thinking about complex problems unconsciously could lead to better solutions than conscious deliberation about the mess that you are in.[38] Allow time for unconscious thought, such as meditation, to help resolve cognitive conflicts, including those associated with broken promises and unkept agreements. Do you know how to meditate? Do you know how to envision a scene that brings you to peace with broken pieces?

But keep in mind the line is subtle and easily gets blurred. The large loops in your subconscious mind created by the accumulation of broken promises and unkept agreements can convince you that you are indeed on the right track. They are never-ending, after all. Remember that one of the primary reasons you break your promises is because you convince yourself that quick rewards are more relevant to you than the long-term perspective.

The enchanted forest wants to keep you in its fold; you are unconsciously addicted to the illusory control it grants you over

[37] Key regulator of decision-making pinpointed in brain, https://medicine.washu.edu/news/key-regulator-of-decision-making-pinpointed-in-brain/

[38] Steindorf L, Rummel J and Boywitt CD (2021) A Fresh Look at the Unconscious Thought Effect: Using Mind-Wandering Measures to Investigate Thought Processes in Decision Problems With High Information Load. *Front. Psychol.* 12:545928. doi: 10.3389/fpsyg.2021.545928

uncertainty. You genuinely believe your impulsive choices can keep us safe. In truth, the enchanted forest is you; it's our common human reality of deep desires seeking to hide from the anxiety and fear that they may never see a tomorrow.

"But wait!" You'll say. "I am smart! I could even be brilliant. I am not the type who falls for illusions." The problem is you do fall for these illusions when you think you don't. Quick rewards convince you they are more relevant to you than the long-term perspective. You sincerely believe that right now, you do have control. You *are* genuinely mastering your conflicts. It is an honest mistake; *you have been living* in the enchanted forest since the inception of humankind and certainly since your creation. How could you ever be wrong?

Have you ever wondered why extraordinary creators have embattled backgrounds, they just can't escape? Why do outstanding artists have torn personal lives and die before their time? At least in a nutshell, the answer is more straightforward than you think: People who show human reality at its most explicit and most direct will exhibit an addiction to the enchanted forest, and not only that, they are more adept than others to dive deeper into this forest and to devise the myriad and one way that will forever also keep them there.

It is through storytelling ~~that~~ you convince yourself that the ways you devise to find your promised gilded path out of the enchanted forest are smart and proper. By nature, you want to stay comfortable so that anything remotely dangerous will not come near you. This includes primarily change, which your brain often perceives as a potential threat[39] since mortal danger can hide behind any rustling in the leaves. So your storytelling ability isn't just for entertainment—it's a crucial survival

[39] Mind Control: How Our Mind Keeps Us Stuck in the Things We Don't Want to Do, by Emmanuel Daniel, https://www.harvestclinic.com.au/post/mind-control-how-our-mind-keeps-us-stuck-in-the-things-we-don-t-want-to-do

mechanism, and yes, it can easily lead you astray. Humans, as a species, are addicted to narration.[40]

At the heart of our narrative-creating ability lies the hippocampus, a seahorse-shaped structure in the brain. The hippocampus is the brain's master storyteller, connecting separate, distant events into a coherent narrative.[41] Interestingly, our brains seem particularly adept at remembering stories related to survival situations. We have better recall for stories involving survival scenarios than other narratives; the most significant effects are when we imagine ourselves as the story character.[42] This "survival processing effect" suggests that our memory systems are fine-tuned to prioritize information that could be crucial for our well-being, but that strategy doesn't necessarily work in our favor!

Our storytelling reflects the vibes of the enchanted forest, especially as these might not accurately reflect reality, but they grant us control and provide our impulses with quick satisfaction; precisely, that dynamic can lend narration its lasting appeal. Our storytelling mind "is allergic to the uncertainty, randomness, and coincidence." It is called on to remedy the very "uncertainty, randomness, and coincidence" that our storytelling mind requires to start to seek its storytelling path. Our storytelling mind "is addicted" to eternally creating meaning.[43]

If you take this tendency to its extreme in your daily life, it can lead your brain to create stories that provide justifications for avoiding situations that make you uncomfortable, even when there is no real danger or when being uncomfortable is a sign of growth. It's a slick mechanism the survival mind employs to keep you in your comfort zone, potentially at the cost of personal growth and new experiences.

---

[40] Gottschall, Jonathan, The Storytelling Animal: How Stories Make Us Human, Mariner Books, 2013.

[41] Hippocampus Is the Brain's Storyteller, by Andy Fell, https://www.ucdavis.edu/health/news/hippocampus-brains-storyteller

[42] Cook, A.M., Klin, C.M. & Westerman, D.L. Surviving with story characters: What do we remember?. *Mem Cogn* 51, 1303–1316 (2023). https://doi.org/10.3758/s13421-022-01391-2

[43] Gottschall, Jonathan, The Storytelling Animal: How Stories Make Us Human, Mariner Books, 2013.

Stories have a special sticking power. When you engage with stories, your brain reacts as if experiencing the events themselves.[44] This phenomenon, linked to mirror neurons, explains why fictional experiences can powerfully impact your emotions and behaviors. The enchanted forest is us, and the stories we tell either keep us in it, addicted to illusory, pleasurable control over anxiety and fear or allow us to transform into the vision we want.

Have you ever found yourself spinning tales of doom and gloom in your head, only to wonder why you're suddenly feeling anxious and afraid? You've probably done so often if you are honest with yourself; in this, you are not alone. You act out the human condition, but only one part of it, the short-term one that brings the immediate gratification you so love to deceive yourself, can be permanent.

Your inner narrator starts with a hefty dose of drama and worst-case scenarios – which can feel good! The self-help language you know refers to this as self-sabotage.[45] Emotional outbursts in negative situations are strangely comforting since you don't see the way out, and being safe feels so good!

So why do you tend to jump to negative conclusions? Your brain is playing a rather clever (albeit annoying) trick on you. When you anticipate potential threats or failures, you're trying to protect yourself by fearing the success you want.[46] Your brain appears to say, "Hey, if I prepare for the worst, I won't be caught off guard!" This self-protective mechanism, while well-intentioned, leads you down a rabbit hole of anxiety and fear.

Recent research in cognitive neuroscience has revealed some intriguing insights into this self-sabotaging behavior:

---

[44] Id.

[45] Bouizegarene N, Ramstead MJD, Constant A, Friston KJ and Kirmayer LJ (2024) Narrative as active inference: an integrative account of cognitive and social functions in adaptation. *Front. Psychol.* 15:1345480. doi: 10.3389/fpsyg.2024.1345480

[46] Self-sabotage: Why it happens and how to overcome it, https://www.medicalnewstoday.com/articles/self-sabotage

1. **Fear Response:** When you conjure up these negative scenarios, your amygdala – the brain's fear center – kicks into high gear. This triggers a stress response, flooding your body with cortisol and preparing you for a fight-or-flight situation. You engage in avoidance behaviors, procrastination, or activities that ensure failure, as these actions can temporarily reduce stress and anxiety by refusing to confront the feared outcome.[47]
2. **Cognitive Dissonance:** Your brain struggles with conflicting beliefs. You might want success but don't feel worthy of it deep down. How could you after all, with a blanket over your head inside the closet? This internal conflict leads to self-sabotaging behaviors to resolve the tension.
3. **Low Self-Esteem:** Individuals with lower self-esteem are more likely to engage in self-sabotage. They confirm their negative self-image; they experience their choices as self-relevant and rewarding.

Awareness of this tendency is the first step towards the change you can bring about as you rewire your mind. Here are a few strategies to help you begin to rewrite your inner narrative:

1. **Recognize the Pattern:** Pay attention to when you start spinning those negative tales.
2. **Challenge Your Thoughts:** When you catch yourself in a self-sabotaging story, pause and ask, "Is this true? What evidence do I have?"
3. **Practice Self-Compassion:** Be kind to yourself. Remember, everyone struggles with self-doubt sometimes.
4. **Focus on the Future:** Try to envision a positive future self. Research shows that feeling connected to your future self can help you make better decisions in the present.[48]

[47] Understanding self-sabotage, https://www.innocentlivesfoundation.org/understanding-self-sabotage/
[48] Self-Sabotage Is Undermining Your Future. Here's How to Conquer It, by Annelise Jolley, January 4th, 2023, https://www.templeton.org/news/self-sabotage

Creatures of anxiety and fear, we all must have our comfort zone – that cozy mental space where everything feels familiar and safe. But here's the thing: your comfort zone can quickly become your prison.[49] Why? Because your visionary, creative self can only grow and change outside of this zone. But your survival-oriented mind resists new choices, preferring the predictable and familiar. Your brain appears to be saying, "Hey, we've survived this long doing things this way, and we've been well and alive; we're even enjoying the enchanted forest. Why rock the boat?" When faced with change, your brain's amygdala – responsible for our fight-or-flight response – lights up like a Christmas tree.[50]

The thought of disturbing the enchanted forest triggers fear and anxiety of what may come at the other end; it's already rustling at you from within the leaves, making you instinctively resist the unknown. Changing that would consume a ton of cognitive energy. When your brain perceives a threat, such as a new situation that might have to be met by a new behavior, it diverts resources away from the prefrontal cortex – the area responsible for rational thinking and decision-making.[51] This makes it harder to process new information and adapt to changes, in turn increasing your anxiety that you are indeed becoming exposed to new threats.

Your brain might be wired for survival rather than thriving, but you're not doomed to stay stuck. The key lies in making new choices consistently over time,[52] and that's a good start. Every time you make a new choice that aligns with your goals, you create new neural pathways in your brain. It's like forging a new trail through the dense forest. The

[49] Mind Control: How Our Mind Keeps Us Stuck in the Things We Don't Want to Do, https://www.harvestclinic.com.au/post/mind-control-how-our-mind-keeps-us-stuck-in-the-things-we-don-t-want-to-do

[50] Neuroscience and L&D: Overcoming Resistance to Change, https://www.sanaross.com/the-neuroscience-of-achieving-more/neuroscience-and-ld-overcoming-resistance-to-change

[51] Id.

[52] Embracing Change: The Neuroscience Behind Thriving in 2024, Insights from Grant Upbeat Bosnick (Chapter 12), https://www.achieveit360.com/embracing-change-the-neuroscience-behind-thriving-in-2024-insights-from-grant-upbeat-bosnick-chapter-12/

first few times are tough, but repetition makes that path more apparent and easier to follow. Here are simple steps that can make it easier:

1. **Start Small**: Break big changes into smaller, less threatening steps. This helps reduce the amygdala's response to fear.
2. **Embrace Discomfort**: Recognize that feeling uncomfortable can be a sign of growth, not danger.
3. **Practice Mindfulness**: This can help you observe your thoughts without getting caught up in them, making it easier to choose new behaviors.[53]
4. **Reframe Change**: Instead of seeing change as a threat, try viewing it as an exciting opportunity for growth and learning.[54]
5. **Be Patient**: Remember, your brain's resistance to change is a feature, not a bug. It takes time to rewire those neural pathways.

These simple steps contain, in a nutshell, a beginning blueprint for growth as a visionary creator. We will take a deep dive into this concept since, as you can imagine, it is not as easy as it sounds. Breaking the chains of human nature's essence since the inception of humankind doesn't come at the snap of your fingers – unless by the snap of your fingers, you mean a trail-blazing, bursting with energy, brand new decision!

There are benefits to completely breaking with the past and adopting a radical change. The good news is that this strategy indeed works – if the new decision is indeed entirely new, bursting with energy, radical and complete. The not-so-good news is that such a decision can still carry the fingerprints of the old world in its wake. You feel better one moment; then the old shows up again – as shadows on the wall, unflushed waste backing up, swelling in the gutter. You feel pain and sadness. You must persist in your decision no matter what!

---

[53] Your mind needs chaos, by Oshan Jarow, October 12, 2024, https://www.vox.com/the-gray-area/376839/creativity-predictive-processing-chaos-mark-miller

[54] Neuroscience and L&D: Overcoming Resistance to Change, https://www.sanaross.com/the-neuroscience-of-achieving-more/neuroscience-and-ld-overcoming-resistance-to-change

As it stands now, these simple steps may not break your chains because these chains are a requirement for you to function daily. Do we want a world where people try to walk out of windows because being the breath of the universe **IS** our true, innermost nature? Of course not! That's why we speak of personal transformation and rewiring our brains instead of radical change.

Awareness is the first concrete step you can take. Understanding your survival mind's storytelling trick is crucial for personal growth and decision-making. By recognizing when your brain might be crafting stories solely to keep you "safe" from perceived threats, pleasurable stories that offer no real way out, you can challenge these narratives and make more informed choices.

As you continue to unravel the mysteries of your storytelling brain, you will gain valuable insights into human cognition and behavior. Your brain's storytelling ability is a remarkable evolutionary adaptation, but it's essential to approach the narratives it creates with a critical eye. By doing so, you can harness the power of your inner storyteller while avoiding the pitfalls of an overzealous survival mind.

Let's embark on the path of consciously crafting more optimistic narratives so you can reshape your brain's patterns and boost your resilience.[55] So, the next time you find yourself weaving a tale of woe, remember: you're the author of your own story. Why not give it a new plot twist that's not a renewed indulgence and illusory while craving control? How can you write a bestseller of hope, growth, and self-compassion instead?

Worrying and seeking immediate but illusory rewards might seem ingrained in your nature, but it's not your destiny. By understanding how

[55] Bouizegarene N, Ramstead MJD, Constant A, Friston KJ and Kirmayer LJ (2024) Narrative as active inference: an integrative account of cognitive and social functions in adaptation. *Front. Psychol.* 15:1345480. doi: 10.3389/fpsyg.2024.1345480

your mind works and consistently making new choices, you can train your brain not just to survive but to thrive. The next time you find yourself resisting change or falling back into old patterns of anxiety and stress, remember your mind might be built for survival, but you have the power to push beyond those limits.

Exercise For Breaking Large, Subconscious Loops

1. Awareness Check
   Ask yourself: "What recurring thought patterns or emotions am I experiencing right now?" Self-awareness is crucial in interrupting unconscious processes
2. Emotional Processing
   Take a deep breath and focus on your body. Where do you feel tension or discomfort? Describe the physical sensations without judgment. Feel your emotions fully.
3. Thought Challenge
   Write down your current thoughts about the situation. Then ask: "Is there any evidence that contradicts these thoughts?" Write down your answers. This question helps challenge automatic thought patterns.
4. Unconscious Integration Period
   Then, set a timer for 5 minutes. During this time, engage in a simple, unrelated task (like solving anagrams or doodling). Complex decisions may benefit from a period of distraction, allowing unconscious processes to integrate information.
5. Conscious Re-evaluation
   After the integration period, revisit your decision. Ask yourself: "Considering all aspects, what feels like the best course of action now?" This final step combines conscious re-evaluation with intuitive feeling, balancing the cognitive and emotional aspects of decision-making.

Both conscious and unconscious processes play roles in effective decision-making.

Exercise to Help With Gloomy Stories You Tell Yourself

1. Identify the Threat Reflex
   What specific aspect of your story triggers your "threat reflex"? Try to pinpoint the exact moment or detail that activates your fear response.
2. Multisensory Engagement
   Describe this moment or detail using all five senses, but with a twist - make each sensory detail slightly absurd or humorous. How does this change your emotional response to the scenario?
3. Engage Top-Down Processing
   How can you reframe the threatening element of your story to make it feel more manageable? Consider alternative perspectives.
4. Stimulate Oxytocin Release
   What elements of trust, connection, or cooperation can you introduce into your story? Focus on aspects that might trigger the release of oxytocin, the "bonding hormone"
5. Creative Network Activation
   Imagine your brain's default network (for spontaneous ideas) collaborating with your executive control network (for focused attention). Create a new story that alternates between free-flowing imagination and structured problem-solving. How does this back-and-forth affect your storytelling process?

THE BENEFITS OF ADDICTION

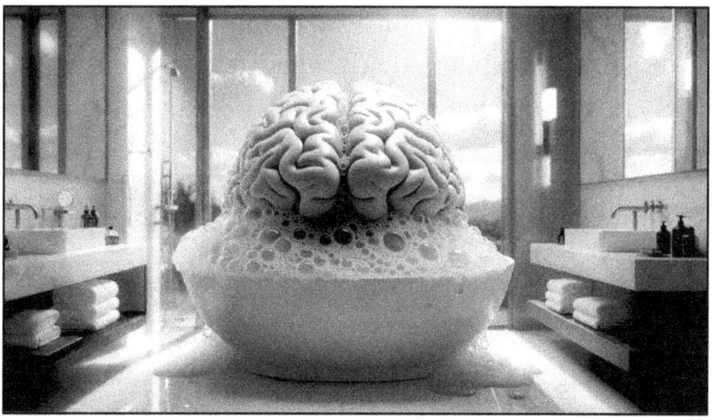

Your brain has an incredible ability to shape your world. However, what you perceive isn't always an accurate representation. You don't see reality. What you see is the story you create. You warp your perceptions to align with your expectations. You bias your perception of time intervals based on prior experiences.[56] This explains why you may feel you complete some tasks faster than what the clock says, while others may take longer. This warping of reality isn't limited to time perception; it affects how you see the world.

[56] How expectation influences perception, https://news.mit.edu/2019/how-expectation-influences-perception-0715

One of the most groundbreaking ideas in modern neuroscience is that our brains are prediction machines. Rather than passively processing incoming sensory information, we constantly predict what we'll experience next. Based on our prior beliefs and experiences, these predictions significantly influence our perception.[57]

Your mind is a remarkable time traveler, constantly peering into the future before it unfolds. Your brain always tries to stay one step ahead of the reality it shapes. Imagine you're watching a friend fly into a rage. Your brain doesn't just process their current emotional state; it's already calculating their likely emotional trajectory. Your brain constantly generates expectations about what's going to happen next.[58] [59] These predictions aren't just limited to social interactions; they apply to virtually every aspect of our perception and cognition.

Your brain does not guess wildly when it makes a prediction. It's using a sophisticated process that involves:

1. Creating internal models based on past experiences;
2. Generating expectations about future states;
3. Comparing these predictions with actual sensory input;
4. Adjusting the models based on any discrepancies (prediction errors).

This process happens automatically and continuously, allowing you to navigate the world more efficiently.[60]

This predictive ability has several advantages. You fill in the gaps in your perceptions, making sense of incomplete information, which is

---

[57] "Reality" is constructed by your brain. Here's what that means, and why it matters, https://www.vox.com/science-and-health/20978285/optical-illusion-science-humility-reality-polarization

[58] Thornton MA, Weaverdyck ME, Tamir DI. The Social Brain Automatically Predicts Others' Future Mental States. J Neurosci. 2019 Jan 2;39(1):140-148. doi: 10.1523/JNEUROSCI.1431-18.2018. Epub 2018 Nov 2. PMID: 30389840; PMCID: PMC6325264.

[59] Mark A Thornton, Diana I Tamir, Perceiving actions before they happen: psychological dimensions scaffold neural action prediction, *Social Cognitive and Affective Neuroscience*, Volume 16, Issue 8, August 2021, Pages 807–815, https://doi.org/10.1093/scan/nsaa126

[60] Bubic A, von Cramon DY, Schubotz RI. Prediction, cognition and the brain. Front Hum Neurosci. 2010 Mar 22;4:25. doi: 10.3389/fnhum.2010.00025. PMID: 20631856; PMCID: PMC2904053.

crucial for threat detection. What would you want to have more than the ability to know when the rustling in the leaves is precisely that, rustling in the leaves, nothing more and nothing less? Predictive mechanisms involve the fear conditioning that will keep you bogged down in illusory control. When fear conditioning occurs, simulations of emotions, or "pre-feelings," may be used to imagine future emotional states,[61] leading to inflexibility, no openness to new experiences, outdated beliefs and biases, and missing out on unexpected opportunities.

Interestingly, your brain does not have to explicitly represent or communicate an expected event to higher cortical areas; those areas have already processed all its relevant features before its occurrence. In contrast, errors of prediction have much greater value. They may signal unsuccessful learning, a significant change in the surroundings, noise, and more minor changes in the body or environment.[62]

By being mindful, curious, challenging assumptions, and embracing uncertainty, you can harness the power of your predictive brain while remaining flexible and adaptable in the face of an ever-changing world. Your mind's ability to predict the future is a double-edged sword. It's a powerful tool that helps you navigate complex social and physical environments. However, it's essential to maintain a balance between leveraging these predictions and remaining open to new possibilities. You have heard the phrase "beyond your wildest dreams." What the future can bring is beyond the predictive abilities of your brain; it can, at best, be the product of your visionary creation.

The predictive nature of the brain explains why it can be so challenging to see new possibilities or change your behaviors. Your brain is wired to confirm your existing beliefs, sometimes even in the face of contradictory evidence. Dr. Joe Dispenza notes, "If we have firm beliefs about something, evidence to the contrary could be sitting right in front

---

[61] Brown EC, Brüne M. The role of prediction in social neuroscience. Front Hum Neurosci. 2012 May 24;6:147. doi: 10.3389/fnhum.2012.00147. PMID: 22654749; PMCID: PMC3359591.

[62] Bubic A, von Cramon DY, Schubotz RI. Prediction, cognition and the brain. Front Hum Neurosci. 2010 Mar 22;4:25. doi: 10.3389/fnhum.2010.00025. PMID: 20631856; PMCID: PMC2904053.

of us, but we may not see it because what we perceive is entirely different."[63] The key lies in understanding that your reality isn't fixed – it's a construct of your brain that you can reshape. Here are ideas to shape your transformation journey:

1. **Challenge Your Beliefs**: Recognize that your beliefs and past experiences influence your perceptions. Actively question your assumptions and seek out new perspectives.
2. **Embrace Neurodiversity**: Remember that each person's brain is as unique as that person's fingerprint. What works for someone else might not work for you, so be open to exploring different approaches to change.
3. **Leverage Neuroplasticity**: Your brain can rewire itself based on new experiences and learning. You can reshape your brain's neural pathways by consistently exposing yourself to new ideas and experiences.[64]
4. **Practice Mindfulness**: Mindfulness meditation can help you become more aware of your thoughts and perceptions. You can recognize when your brain is making assumptions or predictions that may not be accurate.[65]
5. **Visualize New Possibilities**: Use the power of your imagination to visualize new possibilities. This can help create new neural pathways and make it easier for your brain to recognize opportunities in the real world.[66]

But progressing beyond being controlled by how we are wired in the moment is much easier said than done. We crave the cozy satisfaction of the moment much more than we think. We're all familiar with that

[63] Brain fact Friday: Using Neuroscience to Change Our Perception, https://andreasamadi.podbean.com/e/brain-fact-friday-using-neuroscience-to-change-our-perception/

[64] How the brain decides what we perceive, Patterns of brainwaves in the prefrontal cortex gate access to consciousness, April 13, 2023, https://www.mpg.de/20170692/how-the-brain-decides-what-we-perceive

[65] The Neuroscience of Reality, by Anil K. Seth, September 1, 2019, https://www.scientificamerican.com/article/the-neuroscience-of-reality/

[66] "Reality" is constructed by your brain. Here's what that means, and why it matters. By Brian Resnick, January 22, 2020, https://www.vox.com/science-and-health/20978285/optical-illusion-science-humility-reality-polarization

feeling of wanting something badly, whether it's a new job, a relationship, or the latest gadget. Have you ever wondered what's driving those desires? You may be interested in knowing that this wanting game haunts the enchanted forest.

You spend so much time and energy wanting things and trying to achieve your goals. It's as if you constantly search for the next big thing to make you happy. But here's the kicker: your brain isn't always equipped to handle all this wanting and trying as well as you might think.[67] "Incentive salience" or "'wanting'" is a core motivation process in your brain, driven by the brain circuits involving dopamine,[68] the feel-good hormone involved in reward and pleasure, movement, learning and attention, and mood. This 'wanting' differs from our conscious awareness of cognitive desires. It's an unconscious urge that cues in our environment can trigger.[69]

Our 'wanting' system can sometimes go into overdrive, causing us to crave things intensely, even when we don't necessarily enjoy them that much. It's like when you can't stop thinking about that chocolate cake in the fridge, even though you're full and know you won't enjoy eating it.[70] When this system isn't working correctly, it can lead to a lack of motivation and contribute to mental health conditions such as depression and schizophrenia.[71] And when it does work properly, this core

[67] Starita F, Stussi Y, Garofalo S, Terenzi D. Editorial: The neurobiological and cognitive underpinnings of appetitive and aversive motivation. Front Behav Neurosci. 2024 Feb 21;18:1383393. doi: 10.3389/fnbeh.2024.1383393. PMID: 38450023; PMCID: PMC10915259.
[68] Berridge KC, Robinson TE. Liking, wanting, and the incentive-sensitization theory of addiction. Am Psychol. 2016 Nov;71(8):670-679. doi: 10.1037/amp0000059. PMID: 27977239; PMCID: PMC5171207.
[69] Starita F, Stussi Y, Garofalo S, Terenzi D. Editorial: The neurobiological and cognitive underpinnings of appetitive and aversive motivation. Front Behav Neurosci. 2024 Feb 21;18:1383393. doi: 10.3389/fnbeh.2024.1383393. PMID: 38450023; PMCID: PMC10915259.
[70] Berridge KC, Robinson TE. Liking, wanting, and the incentive-sensitization theory of addiction. Am Psychol. 2016 Nov;71(8):670-679. doi: 10.1037/amp0000059. PMID: 27977239; PMCID: PMC5171207.
[71] Starita F, Stussi Y, Garofalo S, Terenzi D. Editorial: The neurobiological and cognitive underpinnings of appetitive and aversive motivation. Front Behav Neurosci. 2024 Feb 21;18:1383393. doi: 10.3389/fnbeh.2024.1383393. PMID: 38450023; PMCID: PMC10915259.

motivation of your brain will be triggered by the rustling in the leaves, causing you to crave that habitual, illusory control intensely. As a healthy person, you know to rewire your brain so as not to get stuck with the creations of your anxieties and fears.

As you may now be suspecting, deep down, fear is a primary motivator for many of our actions.[72] Even when we think we're pursuing positive goals, an underlying current of fear is often driving us. This fear can take many forms. It might be fear of missing out, fear of failure, or fear of success. Your brain constantly looks for potential threats, even when going after something you want[73] - especially then.

So next time you find yourself caught up in the wanting game, take a deep breath and remember: your brain is doing its best to navigate a complex world. Be kind to yourself, and stay curious about your motivations. Who knows? You might just find that what you wanted was inside you all along.

Being stuck in a cycle of self-relevant, strangely rewarding but negative thoughts, unable to break free, is more than just a frustrating experience - it's a form of addiction to your thoughts and emotions. Your brain is incredibly adaptable, constantly forming new neural connections based on your thoughts and experiences. This neuroplasticity allows you to learn and grow throughout your life. However, it also means you can inadvertently "train" your brain to fall into specific emotional patterns. You strengthen the neural pathways associated with those mental states when you repeatedly think specific thoughts or experience particular emotions. Over time, these pathways become your default mode of thinking and feeling, creating what neuroscientists call "emotional habits."[74]

---

[72] Berridge KC (2018) Evolving Concepts of Emotion and Motivation. *Front. Psychol.* 9:1647. doi: 10.3389/fpsyg.2018.01647

[73] Id.

[74] Addiction study reveals distinct cognitive mechanisms behind different behaviors, https://www.psypost.org/addiction-study-reveals-distinct-cognitive-mechanisms-behind-different-behaviors/

You wake up each morning in the same emotional state, repeating the same thoughts, which leads to the same behaviors.[75] Have you ever woken up in the morning with a dislike of a person or situation, no matter how fleeting? Did you find yourself in similar circumstances during the day as you had wanted to move away from in the past? The causation does not have to be direct, but there is usually a correlation! Spend some time reflecting on this; you're now discovering why you experience this predicament.

The mechanisms behind these emotional habits share similarities with those involved in substance addictions. Distinct cognitive processes drive different types of addictive behaviors, including thought patterns. Reward-related neurocognitive processes play a crucial role in various non-substance-related addictive behaviors. These processes manifest differently depending on the specific behavior in question.[76]

Your ability to regulate emotions is a key factor in the formation of emotional habits so that you can break the cycle of fear. The brain regulates emotions; we separate emotion regulation from activity related to emotion generation.[77] Emotion regulation, or "reappraisal," involves particular areas of the anterior prefrontal cortex. These regions are crucial for abstract thought and long-term representations of the future. Interestingly, the more you activate these emotion-regulation brain regions, the more resilient you are to negative experiences. Being resilient to adverse experiences can generate non-negative emotions. This suggests that strengthening your emotion regulation skills could help break negative thought patterns.[78]

---

[75] How to stop living on autopilot, https://www.yourcabana.com/blog/how-to-stop-living-on-autopilot

[76] Addiction study reveals distinct cognitive mechanisms behind different behaviors, by Eric W. Dolan, September 3, 2024, https://www.psypost.org/addiction-study-reveals-distinct-cognitive-mechanisms-behind-different-behaviors/

[77] "Researchers map how the brain regulates emotions." ScienceDaily, 3 April 2024. www.sciencedaily.com/releases/2024/04/240403170916.htm

[78] "Researchers map how the brain regulates emotions." ScienceDaily. ScienceDaily, 3 April 2024. www.sciencedaily.com/releases/2024/04/240403170916.htm

Long-term representations of the future play a crucial role in emotion regulation. Is where you see your emotions leading you beneficial in the long term? Can you reconcile your current emotional state with your ideal version of yourself? These are two impactful questions to help you with emotion regulation.

And emotion regulation is not enough. Habits are shaped by two brain systems: one that triggers automatic responses to familiar cues and another that enables goal-directed control. The imbalance between these two systems can lead to compulsive behaviors or thought patterns. Habits happen when automatic responses outweigh your ability to consciously control them,[79] which explains once more why illusory control in the enchanted forest can be such a pleasurably sticking habit. It's your habit of automatic, compulsive responses with quick rewards.

A single belief disturbance can trigger and maintain compulsive behavior, such as a lack of confidence in the effectiveness of your preventive actions.[80] Have you ever found yourself scrolling through social media when you should be doing something else or reaching for a snack even though you're not hungry? If you don't trust that you can effectively control a situation, you are more likely to engage in repetitive, compulsive behaviors.

You need to tip the balance back towards goal-directed control. Goal-directed behavior, especially with long-term representations of the future, is beneficial in regulating your emotions and keeping them away from automatic, potentially compulsive actions. You can achieve this through strategies such as implementation intentions, which happen when you envision, "If situation X occurs, then I will do Y."

---

[79] Cognitive neuroscientists discover new blueprint for making and breaking habits, https://medicalxpress.com/news/2024-11-cognitive-neuroscientists-blueprint-habits.html

[80] Rigoux L, Stephan KE, Petzschner FH. Beliefs, compulsive behavior and reduced confidence in control. PLoS Comput Biol. 2024 Jun 20;20(6):e1012207. doi: 10.1371/journal.pcbi.1012207. PMID: 38900828; PMCID: PMC11218963.

Here is a playbook for behavior change that connects brain science with practical, real-world applications:[81]

1. Implementation intentions: Creating "if-then" plans to guide our responses in specific situations.
2. Exposure therapy: Gradually facing fears to reduce automatic anxiety responses.
3. Habit reversal therapy: Replacing unwanted habits with more beneficial behaviors.

Emotion regulation plays a critical role in healing from addiction and compulsive behaviors.[82] Improving your ability to regulate emotions could be key to breaking free from the wanting game and the negative thought patterns and emotional habits that come with it. You can rewire your brain for greater emotional resilience and well-being with practice and persistence. After all, if you can invest the effort to become addicted to your thoughts, you can also learn to direct them towards more positive, forward-looking paths.

Have you ever felt stuck in a loop, repeating the same emotional patterns daily? You're not alone. Many people find themselves trapped in "living on autopilot." Recent cognitive neuroscience research has highlighted why we often find ourselves in this autopilot state. Our brains have developed a subconscious system to handle routine tasks, decisions, and thoughts with little cognitive effort. This system, known as the default mode network (DMN), allows us to perform tasks quickly and accurately without conscious thought.[83] While this autopilot mode can

---

[81] Cognitive neuroscientists discover new blueprint for making and breaking habits, by Fiona Tyrrell, November 19, 2024, https://medicalxpress.com/news/2024-11-cognitive-neuroscientists-blueprint-habits.html#google_vignette

[82] Hand, L.J., Paterson, L.M. & Lingford-Hughes, A.R. Re-evaluating our focus in addiction: emotional dysregulation is a critical driver of relapse to drug use. *Transl Psychiatry* **14**, 467 (2024). https://doi.org/10.1038/s41398-024-03159-5

[83] Your autopilot mode is real - now we know how the brain does it, https://www.newscientist.com/article/2151137-your-autopilot-mode-is-real-now-we-know-how-the-brain-does-it/

benefit routine tasks, it can limit our growth and harm our overall well-being when we allow it to dominate our emotional lives.[84]

Emotional autopilot refers to the automatic response patterns based on absolutes or learned behaviors. You might find yourself answering "fine" or "tired" when asked how you are without assessing your current emotional state. You might say, “I am off to work,” just because it is 8 a.m. This disconnection from your genuine emotions can lead to detachment, indifference, and a sense of watching life pass by rather than actively participating.

Interestingly, dopamine or “feel good” production in the brain can explain your vulnerability to these automatic behaviors. Short-term memory capacity also plays a role in our susceptibility to autopilot behaviors.[85] But your tendency to fall into emotional routines isn't entirely automatic and can be controlled. This is an essential insight since so much of our modern lives are lived according to routines. Your mode of transportation and daily routes to work, for example, tasks for your profession you must complete, or how you like to spend the holidays. Now you know why what you engage in with all good intentions can lead to burnout, dissatisfaction, anxiety, and a dreaded loss of meaning.

You can snap out of this emotional autopilot and live more intentionally. Here are some strategies:

1. **Practice Mindfulness**: Mindfulness affects your brain's amygdala, which regulates your body's stress response. You can balance your emotional reactions by actively working to be present in the moment instead of being a participant on autopilot.[86]
2. **Engage Your Intentional System**: Your brain has two thinking systems - the autopilot system and the intentional system. By consciously engaging our intentional system centered in the

---

[84] How to stop living on autopilot, https://www.yourcabana.com/blog/how-to-stop-living-on-autopilot
[85] Living on autopilot: the role of dopamine, By Ping Chen, 24 March 2023, https://blog.donders.ru.nl/?lang=en&p=14951
[86] Id.

prefrontal cortex, you can override habitual behaviors and make more deliberate choices.[87]

3. **Challenge Your Routines**: Introduce small changes to your daily routine to jolt yourself out of autopilot. This could be as simple as taking a different route to work or trying a new hobby.
4. **Regular Self-Assessment**: Take time each day to honestly assess your emotional state. This self-awareness can help you recognize when you're slipping into autopilot mode.
5. **Train Your Brain**: Just as you can train your body, you can also train your brain. Over time, you can use your intentional system to change your automatic thinking, feeling, and behavior patterns.[88]

Breaking free from emotional autopilot is a process. It requires consistent effort and patience. However, the rewards are significant. Living more intentionally allows you to experience greater emotional richness, make decisions that align with your goals, and ultimately lead a more fulfilling life. So, the next time you wake up, take a moment to check in with yourself. Are you repeating yesterday's emotional state, or are you ready to write a new emotional script for the day? The choice is more in your hands than you might think.

Stress plays a crucial role in your emotional addiction. Stress is a complex physiological and psychological response to perceived threats or challenges.[89] It involves the activation of neuroendocrine systems, primarily the HPA axis that controls the release of hormones and the SAM that mediates short-term effects, producing rapid responses. [90] Unlike fear, which is an immediate alarm response, or anxiety, which is

[87] Korponay C. Snapping Out of Autopilot: Overriding Habits in Real Time and the Role of Ventrolateral Prefrontal Cortex. Perspect Psychol Sci. 2023 Mar;18(2):482-490. doi: 10.1177/17456916221120033. Epub 2022 Sep 22. PMID: 36137178; PMCID: PMC10023494.

[88] Autopilot vs. Intentional System: The Rider and the Elephant, https://intentionalinsights.org/autopilot-vs-intentional-system-the-rider-and-the-elephant/

[89] Valencia-Florez KB, Sánchez-Castillo H, Vázquez P, Zarate P, Paz DB. Stress, a Brief Update. Int J Psychol Res (Medellin). 2023 Oct 10;16(2):105-121. doi: 10.21500/20112084.5815. PMID: 38106958; PMCID: PMC10723744.

[90] Id.

an anticipatory response, stress is an ongoing process that can encompass both, potentially leading to adaptive behaviors that can be unfavorable and, if chronic, lead to various health issues.[91] [92]

Breaking free from stress addiction can be a challenging journey, especially when you've grown accustomed to a high-stress lifestyle. Imagine waking up one morning feeling unusually calm and relaxed. This newfound tranquility might feel foreign and even unsettling for someone chronically stressed. You'll mentally grab for any next best thing just to make you feel stressed again. Let's explore what happens in your brain during this process and why you might unconsciously seek stress to feel "normal" again.

Stress fundamentally changes your memories and cognitive processes. Stress alters how your brain encodes and retrieves aversive memories.[93] When you are under stress, your brain forms larger, more generalized memory engrams – physical representations of memories in the brain. These expanded engrams can lead to the generalization of fearful memories, similar to what occurs in post-traumatic stress disorder (PTSD). You find yourself surrounded by a gloomy mood.

Interestingly, stress doesn't always impair memory formation. Cortisol, a key stress hormone, can enhance memory encoding for emotional experiences.[94] This explains why you have vivid recollections of stressful events. However, there's a catch – while individual elements of stressful episodes are remembered more clearly, the connections

---

[91] Hofmann SG, Ellard KK, Siegle GJ. Neurobiological correlates of cognitions in fear and anxiety: a cognitive-neurobiological information-processing model. Cogn Emot. 2012;26(2):282-99. doi: 10.1080/02699931.2011.579414. Epub 2011 Aug 1. PMID: 21806384; PMCID: PMC3229257.

[92] Sarmiento LF, Lopes da Cunha P, Tabares S, Tafet G, Gouveia A Jr. Decision-making under stress: A psychological and neurobiological integrative model. Brain Behav Immun Health. 2024 Apr 16;38:100766. doi: 10.1016/j.bbih.2024.100766. PMID: 38694793; PMCID: PMC11061251.

[93] "How stress is fundamentally changing our memories." ScienceDaily. ScienceDaily, 15 November 2024. www.sciencedaily.com/releases/2024/11/241115124541.htm

[94] Stress Amplifies the Brain's Ability to Encode Memory, New Study Finds, by Isabella Backman, https://medicine.yale.edu/news-article/stress-amplifies-the-brains-ability-to-encode-memory-new-study-finds/

between these elements may be weaker. You may be at a loss in making sense of your stressful responses. Stress can also impact your cognitive reserve, which is the brain's ability to cope with damage and maintain function. While mentally stimulating activities can improve cognition, high stress levels undermine this beneficial relationship and deplete you.[95]

When you wake up feeling calm after a period of chronic stress, your brain might struggle to adjust to this new state. Here's what you could experience:

1. **Memory Retrieval**: Your brain is accustomed to stress and might automatically retrieve memories of past stressful experiences.[96] This could trigger feelings of anxiety or unease.
2. **Cortisol Craving**: Your body, used to higher cortisol levels, might signal for more stress to feel "normal."[97]
3. **Cognitive Dissonance**: The calm state might feel so unfamiliar that your mind interprets it as something being wrong, prompting a return to stress.[98]
4. **Stress-Seeking Behavior**: You might unconsciously seek out stressful situations or create stress to return to your familiar state.

Overcoming stress addiction requires rewiring your brain's response to the calm states that feel unusual to you. Here are some strategies:

1. **Mindfulness Practice**: Regular meditation can help reduce cortisol levels and improve cognition.[99]

---

[95] "How stress knocks out your cognitive reserve." ScienceDaily. ScienceDaily, 4 June 2024. www.sciencedaily.com/releases/2024/06/240604132046.htm

[96] "How stress is fundamentally changing our memories." ScienceDaily. ScienceDaily, 15 November 2024. www.sciencedaily.com/releases/2024/11/241115124541.htm

[97] Stress Amplifies the Brain's Ability to Encode Memory, New Study Finds, by Isabella Backman, https://medicine.yale.edu/news-article/stress-amplifies-the-brains-ability-to-encode-memory-new-study-finds/

[98] "How stress knocks out your cognitive reserve." ScienceDaily. ScienceDaily, 4 June 2024. www.sciencedaily.com/releases/2024/06/240604132046.htm

[99] Karolinska Institutet. "How stress knocks out your cognitive reserve." ScienceDaily, 4 June 2024. www.sciencedaily.com/releases/2024/06/240604132046.htm

2. **Create New Positive Memories**: Engage in enjoyable, low-stress activities to form new, positive memory engrams.[100]
3. **Cognitive Restructuring**: Work on reframing your perception of calm as a positive state rather than a cause for concern.
4. **Gradual Exposure**: Slowly increase periods of calm in your day to help your brain adjust.

Remember, just as your brain adapted to chronic stress, it can adapt to a calmer lifestyle. It is up to you to make the switch.

Exercise to Break The Autopilot Craving Cycle

1. Awareness Check:
   Take a moment to pause and scan your body. On a scale of 1-5, how intense is your current craving? What physical sensations do you notice? Write down your responses.
2. Trigger Identification:
   What environmental cues or emotional states preceded this craving? Try to identify at least one external (e.g., location, smell, image) and one internal (e.g., stress, boredom) trigger. Write these down.
3. Cognitive Reappraisal:
   How can you reframe your thoughts about the craved item or experience? Generate at least two alternative perspectives that align with your long-term health goals. Write this down.
4. Value-Based Decision Making:
   Visualize your future self who has successfully managed this craving. What positive outcomes do you anticipate? How do the positive outcomes align with your personal values? Write a clear paragraph of your story.

---

[100] The Hospital for Sick Children. "How stress is fundamentally changing our memories." ScienceDaily, 15 November 2024. www.sciencedaily.com/releases/2024/11/241115124541.htm

5. Regulation Strategy:
   Based on your responses, choose one action to take right now that can help regulate your emotional state and reduce the craving intensity. This could be a brief mindfulness exercise, physical activity, or engaging in a personally meaningful task.

After completing this exercise, reassess your craving intensity on the 1-5 scale. Notice any changes in your physical sensations or emotional state. Remember, consistent practice of these questions can strengthen the neural pathways associated with emotion regulation. Over time, this can help shift your brain from autopilot responses to more intentional, goal-directed behaviors.

THE MIRACLE THAT IS YOU

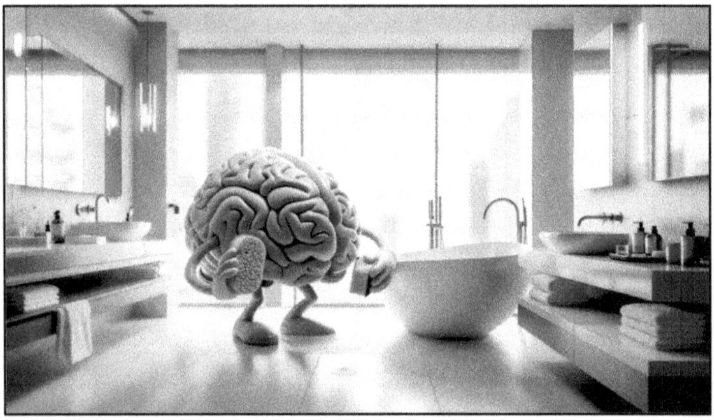

How you perceive the external world is emerging as the crux of transformative experience. Here, we speak about how, by transforming your perception of this world, you can change your daily life experiences. It is insightful to note that a simple walk in nature can influence your resting brain activity. Specifically, a simple walk in nature affects a neural oscillation called the Frontal Midline Theta (FMθ), associated with executive attention and deep relaxation.[101]

[101] Id.

And that's not all this crucial brain rhythm does. It reflects sustained attention during various cognitive tasks and skilled performances.[102] FMθ activity increases during:[103]

- Mental calculations and arithmetic tasks;
- Psychological tasks requiring attention;
- Preparation for skilled actions (e.g., [deleted] golf putting);
- Driving tasks;[104]
- Meditation states.[105]

FMθ signals have been linked to anxiety and cognitive control mechanisms, indicating that FMθ can reflect a common mechanism for implementing adaptive control in uncertain situations.[106]

The Default Mode Network (DMN) is a set of brain regions that become active when you are not focused on the external world. It's associated with self-referential thinking, mind-wandering, and memory retrieval.[107] Urban environments are associated with reduced volume in a key part of the DMN, the medial prefrontal cortex, decreased functional

---

[102] Kao SC, Huang CJ, Hung TM. Frontal midline theta is a specific indicator of optimal attentional engagement during skilled putting performance. J Sport Exerc Psychol. 2013 Oct;35(5):470-8. doi: 10.1123/jsep.35.5.470. PMID: 24197715.

[103] Interestingly, lower FMθ power has been associated with optimal attentional engagement and successful skilled performance. In a study on golf putting, decreased FMθ power was observed during participants' best putts compared to their worst putts, suggesting that excessive attentional control may not always be beneficial. See the discussion on intuition later in this book. Kao SC, Huang CJ, Hung TM. Frontal midline theta is a specific indicator of optimal attentional engagement during skilled putting performance. J Sport Exerc Psychol. 2013 Oct;35(5):470-8. doi: 10.1123/jsep.35.5.470. PMID: 24197715.

[104] Ueno K, Ishii R, Ueda M, Yuri T, Shiroma C, Hata M and Naito Y (2023) Frontal midline theta rhythm and gamma activity measured by sheet-type wearable EEG device. *Front. Hum. Neurosci.* 17:1145282. doi: 10.3389/fnhum.2023.1145282

[105] Ishii R, Canuet L, Ishihara T, Aoki Y, Ikeda S, Hata M, Katsimichas T, Gunji A, Takahashi H, Nakahachi T, Iwase M, Takeda M. Frontal midline theta rhythm and gamma power changes during focused attention on mental calculation: an MEG beamformer analysis. Front Hum Neurosci. 2014 Jun 11;8:406. doi: 10.3389/fnhum.2014.00406. PMID: 24966825; PMCID: PMC4052629.

[106] Cavanagh JF, Shackman AJ. Frontal midline theta reflects anxiety and cognitive control: meta-analytic evidence. J Physiol Paris. 2015 Feb-Jun;109(1-3):3-15. doi: 10.1016/j.jphysparis.2014.04.003. Epub 2014 Apr 29. PMID: 24787485; PMCID: PMC4213310.

[107] Raffone, A., Srinivasan, N. Mindfulness and Cognitive Functions: Toward a Unifying Neurocognitive Framework. *Mindfulness* **8**, 1–9 (2017). https://doi.org/10.1007/s12671-016-0654-1

connectivity within this network, and dysregulation in stress processing.[108] On the other hand, mindfulness training can lead to changes in brain structure and function, particularly in areas associated with attention, emotion regulation, and self-awareness.[109]

By practicing mindfulness, we become aware of how, by transforming our perception of the world, we can change the world as we see it. It starts with basic steps. That person that so annoys you who may be passing by any minute? But there is a book or any object adjacent to where that horror will be, an object that you enjoy so much – your fascination is wholly absorbed by it. What will you do with that book or object just now? Try such simple tricks, and you'll be amazed at how your world can change.

By being mindful of this transformation, you can make informed choices about how you choose to perceive your surroundings to support your cognitive well-being and personal growth. You must make this choice consciously so that you can create new neural pathways and expand your cognitive horizons. Strictly speaking, there is no need to live in nature, but you should use caution when training yourself to transform how you perceive the outside world. Have you heard the phrase that you shouldn't listen to meditation tapes while driving? Meditation activates circuits in your brain that are very different from autopilot mode.

Have you had that moment when you suddenly become aware of your own existence? That instant when you experience you've awakened from a dream, even though you are already awake? This fascinating phenomenon is closely tied to our understanding of consciousness and self-awareness. Recent advancements in cognitive neuroscience have shed new light on this experience of "awakening" or becoming self-aware. We

[108] Polemiti, E., Hese, S., Schepanski, K. *et al.* How does the macroenvironment influence brain and behaviour—a review of current status and future perspectives. *Mol Psychiatry* **29**, 3268–3286 (2024). https://doi.org/10.1038/s41380-024-02557-x

[109] Weder BJ. Mindfulness in the focus of the neurosciences - The contribution of neuroimaging to the understanding of mindfulness. Front Behav Neurosci. 2022 Oct 17;16:928522. doi: 10.3389/fnbeh.2022.928522. PMID: 36325155; PMCID: PMC9622333.

can now map the intricate brain networks that contribute to conscious self-awareness with unprecedented detail.[110]

A subcortical brain network is crucial for integrating arousal and awareness in human consciousness. This network, dubbed the "default ascending arousal network," sustains wakefulness in the resting, conscious human brain. Pathways connecting various brain parts, including the brainstem, thalamus, hypothalamus, basal forebrain, and cerebral cortex, form a complex web that keeps you awake and aware.[111]

Self-awareness, or the ability to recognize oneself as the object of one's thoughts, is a key component of consciousness. It's believed to be an emergent property observed at different levels of cognitive complexity.[112] Self-awareness relies on several bodily experiences, including:

- Self-location (where you perceive your body to be in space);
- Body ownership (the feeling that your body belongs to you);
- Agency (the sense that you're in control of your actions);
- First-person perspective (seeing the world from your viewpoint).[113]

Interoceptive signals, or the perception of your bodily sensations, likely contribute significantly to your sense of self and consciousness.[114]

We must approach understanding consciousness from a perspective of world transformation and new world-building. You can transform how

---

[110] "Brain imaging study reveals connections critical to human consciousness." ScienceDaily. ScienceDaily, 1 May 2024. www.sciencedaily.com/releases/2024/05/240501152947.htm

[111] Massachusetts General Hospital. "Brain imaging study reveals connections critical to human consciousness." ScienceDaily, 1 May 2024. www.sciencedaily.com/releases/2024/05/240501152947.htm

[112] Mograbi DC, Hall S, Arantes B, Huntley J. The cognitive neuroscience of self-awareness: Current framework, clinical implications, and future research directions. Wiley Interdiscip Rev Cogn Sci. 2024 Mar-Apr;15(2):e1670. doi: 10.1002/wcs.1670. Epub 2023 Dec 3. PMID: 38043919.

[113] Understanding the neural bases of bodily self-consciousness: recent achievements and main challenges, Front. Integr. Neurosci., 18 June 2023, Volume 17 - 2023 | https://doi.org/10.3389/fnint.2023.1145924

[114] Dary Z and Lopez C (2023) Understanding the neural bases of bodily self-consciousness: recent achievements and main challenges. *Front. Integr. Neurosci.* 17:1145924. doi: 10.3389/fnint.2023.1145924

you see the world and become a creator instead of an impulse chaser. Researchers can observe brain activity associated with conscious experiences, but interpreting this data and understanding how it relates to our subjective experiences is the responsibility of each of us individually. Science can manipulate thoughts, perceptions, and emotions but cannot penetrate human awareness completely.

In the words of one scientist, "Our ability to measure things far outstrips our ability to understand what we're measuring."[115] Know this: you share the energy networks that support your body and mind with the energy that supports the universe; that energy continuously moves, transforms, and expands, as can be exemplified by many meditation and psychological practices. You have awareness, or a sense of a broader self, even when you are unconscious and unaware of yourself.

This all-encompassing awareness can be put to good use in daily life. Metacognition is often described as "thinking about thinking;" it enables self-reflection and cognitive control. The interplay of metacognition and awareness plays a crucial role in shaping your mental landscape and influencing your ability to navigate challenges with resilience and foresight. These two processes work together to lay the foundation for mental calm and a visionary mindset.

Self-awareness focuses on understanding the "what" and "why" of your experiences, while meta-knowledge involves understanding the "how" of your thought processes. Meta-knowledge contributes to self-regulation abilities. You recognize and monitor your mental states, understand your cognitive processes, including your thoughts about thoughts, emotions about emotions, and beliefs about beliefs. This helps you adjust your behavior accordingly.[116] Both meta-knowledge and self-

[115] From AI to optogenetics, new techniques and strategies are enabling researchers to learn from cognitive disorders and probe the root of consciousness, https://cifar.ca/publications-reports/reach/how-does-the-brain-give-rise-to-the-mind/

[116] Self Awareness and Meta Awareness, by Sid Khullar, July 29, 2023, https://raashealth.in/2023/07/29/self-awareness-and-meta-awareness/#

awareness are components of metacognition and reflection, which plays a critical role in learning and personal growth.[117]

Metacognition enables you to regulate your learning strategies effectively and make more informed decisions. Metacognition, or "thinking about thinking," involves two key components: knowledge of cognition and regulation of cognition.[118] [119] The brain regions associated with metacognitive processes work in concert to enable self-reflection and cognitive control,[120] such as planning and adapting behavior based on outcomes. These processes can overlap with meta-knowledge. Metacognitive judgments of confidence, or subjective evaluations of your cognitive processes, reflect the degree of certainty in the accuracy of your decisions, memories, or predictions.[121]

The pervasive, aware, reflective power of your meta-cognition brings meta-control into the awareness you apply in your daily life. Your domain-specific meta-knowledge processes select, adapt, and correct your cognitive strategies; they guide you as you use your cognitive control, apply judgments of conscience and evaluations, and plan and adjust your behavior.[122] You align your confidence levels with your performance, reducing overconfidence in wrong decisions. You recognize mistakes even without explicit feedback, preventing repeated errors.[123]

---

[117] Self-Awareness: The Power of Metacognition in Education, https://futureeducationmagazine.com/metacognition-in-education/

[118] Balconi M, Acconito C, Allegretta RA, Crivelli D. What Is the Relationship between Metacognition and Mental Effort in Executive Functions? The Contribution of Neurophysiology. Behav Sci (Basel). 2023 Nov 10;13(11):918. doi: 10.3390/bs13110918. PMID: 37998665; PMCID: PMC10669885.

[119] Fleur, D.S., Bredeweg, B. & van den Bos, W. Metacognition: ideas and insights from neuro- and educational sciences. *npj Sci. Learn.* **6**, 13 (2021). https://doi.org/10.1038/s41539-021-00089-5

[120] Cognitive neuroscience—the awareness of ignorance, by Juntendo University, January 26, 2018, https://medicalxpress.com/news/2018-01-cognitive-neurosciencethe-awareness.html

[121] Fleur, D.S., Bredeweg, B. & van den Bos, W. Metacognition: ideas and insights from neuro- and educational sciences. *npj Sci. Learn.* **6**, 13 (2021). https://doi.org/10.1038/s41539-021-00089-5

[122] Jia X, Li W and Cao L (2019) The Role of Metacognitive Components in Creative Thinking. *Front. Psychol.* 10:2404. doi: 10.3389/fpsyg.2019.02404

[123] Yeung N, Summerfield C. Metacognition in human decision-making: confidence and error monitoring. Philos Trans R Soc Lond B Biol Sci. 2012 May 19;367(1594):1310-21. doi: 10.1098/rstb.2011.0416. PMID: 22492749; PMCID: PMC3318764.

So when something appears spiritual and apparently uplifting but somewhat abstract and meaningless to you, it could precisely be that. You did not apply and use the strategies that your meta-knowledge created! Which means you likely did not use any meta-cognitive control. Your actions were devoid of your spirit. Knowledge without doing is dead knowledge.

What happens when you bring meta-cognition and -control into the awareness you apply in your daily life decisions? You have the power of change. There is a moment when, recognizing and monitoring your mental states, you decide to adjust and change your behavior. You gain certainty in the accuracy of your decisions, memories, or predictions; you are genuinely self-aware. Metacognition helps create these subjective experiences of conscious presence. ~40Hz Gamma oscillations, heightened awareness, deep focus, sharp mental clarity, and dopamine become instrumental in generating self-awareness.[124] It is interesting to note that experienced meditators exhibit high levels of gamma synchrony during meditation sessions. It is by accurately doing, reflecting on and changing or correcting ourselves that we are most 'meditatively' or most precisely and clearly self-aware.

Self-awareness and cognitive regulation can seamlessly align. As explicit self-awareness decreases, you can experience an increased sense of control over the task at hand.[125] You achieve heightened states of consciousness in your performance.

You may have observed how some people execute decision-making tasks on the fly, at a rapid pace, without the *need* to reflect on their actions

---

[124] Lou HC, Changeux JP, Rosenstand A. Towards a cognitive neuroscience of self-awareness. Neurosci Biobehav Rev. 2017 Dec;83:765-773. doi: 10.1016/j.neubiorev.2016.04.004. Epub 2016 Apr 11. PMID: 27079562.

[125] Gold J, Ciorciari J. A Review on the Role of the Neuroscience of Flow States in the Modern World. Behav Sci (Basel). 2020 Sep 9;10(9):137. doi: 10.3390/bs10090137. PMID: 32916878; PMCID: PMC7551835.

to perform them.[126] You may well have yourself engaged in such tasks. Your metacognitive processes are crucial in learning, decision-making, and self-awareness. The prefrontal cortex, particularly its anterior and lateral portions, is a key player in metacognitive processes. This area seems especially important for the accuracy of retrospective judgments about your performance.[127] You can productively use these judgments when you engage in essential tasks.

The mindful awareness you put to use daily when you make confident, accurate decisions works synergistically with metacognition to create a calm state. Mindfulness meditation can enhance metacognitive abilities, improve emotional regulation, and reduce stress.[128] Mindfulness practice increases awareness of thoughts and feelings in the present moment, allowing for a more objective observation of mental processes then when we must decide to be confident, to observe and correct ourselves, to make a proactive, forward-looking change. Regular mindfulness practice strengthens neural connections related to emotional control, particularly in the dorsolateral prefrontal cortex. This strengthening of executive control functions enables you to manage emotional responses and maintain a sense of calm in the face of challenges.

The combination of heightened awareness and strong metacognitive skills contributes to developing a visionary mindset. Underlying this is your ability to reflect on and evaluate your mental states and skills and assess your thoughts, emotions, and behaviors[129] so you can foresee and adapt to changes.

---

[126] Fleur, D.S., Bredeweg, B. & van den Bos, W. Metacognition: ideas and insights from neuro- and educational sciences. *npj Sci. Learn.* **6**, 13 (2021). https://doi.org/10.1038/s41539-021-00089-5

[127] Fleming SM, Dolan RJ. The neural basis of metacognitive ability. Philos Trans R Soc Lond B Biol Sci. 2012 May 19;367(1594):1338-49. doi: 10.1098/rstb.2011.0417. PMID: 22492751; PMCID: PMC3318765.

[128] Metacognition: The Key to Self-Awareness and Resilience, August 25, 2024, https://resiliencei.com/blog/metacognition-the-key-to-self-awareness-and-resilience

[129] Yunxuan Zheng, Samuel Recht, Dobromir Rahnev, Common computations for metacognition and meta-metacognition, *Neuroscience of Consciousness*, Volume 2023, Issue 1, 2023, niad023, https://doi.org/10.1093/nc/niad023

The involvement of the anterior prefrontal cortex in metacognitive sensitivity, particularly in perception-related tasks, suggests that improving metacognitive abilities may enhance your capacity to perceive and interpret complex information,[130] a crucial skill for developing a forward-thinking, visionary perspective.

Cognitive neuroscience suggests several strategies so you can harness the power of awareness and metacognition for mental calm and visionary thinking:

1. **Practice Self-Reflection**: Regular self-reflection enhances metacognitive skills by increasing awareness of thought patterns and decision-making processes.
2. **Engage in Mindful Meditation**: Mindfulness practices strengthen the neural pathways associated with emotional regulation and cognitive control.
3. **Slow Down Thinking**: Taking time to consider decisions allows for more thorough metacognitive processing, reducing biases and improving decision quality.
4. **Seek Feedback**: External input provides valuable perspectives that enhance metacognitive awareness and improve cognitive strategies.[131]
5. **Attention Training**: Techniques that improve attention flexibility can enhance metacognitive control and reduce rumination.[132]

By implementing these practices, you cultivate a state of mental calm that serves as a foundation for visionary thinking. The enhanced awareness and metacognitive skills allow for better management of

---

[130] Fleur, D.S., Bredeweg, B. & van den Bos, W. Metacognition: ideas and insights from neuro- and educational sciences. *npj Sci. Learn.* **6**, 13 (2021). https://doi.org/10.1038/s41539-021-00089-5

[131] Metacognition: The Key to Self-Awareness and Resilience, August 25, 2024, https://resiliencei.com/blog/metacognition-the-key-to-self-awareness-and-resilience

[132] Metacognition: Dangerous or Hidden Key to Mental Resilience? https://metacognitivetherapycentral.com/metacognition-dangerous-or-hidden-key-to-mental-resilience/

cognitive resources, enabling a more balanced and forward-looking approach to challenges and opportunities. Understanding and leveraging this enhances your ability to navigate complex mental landscapes and maintain emotional equilibrium, which is essential in today's rapidly changing world.

When you make decisions, you often focus solely on what you want to do or achieve. However, this approach overlooks a crucial aspect of decision-making: the cognitive processes that shape your choices and ultimately determine your results.[133]

Decision-making is a complex interplay between different brain regions, particularly the prefrontal cortex and the hippocampus. These areas work together to simulate potential outcomes and guide your choices based on past experiences and future goals. One of the key findings in recent cognitive neuroscience is the importance of mental simulation in decision-making. When you pause to think before making an important decision, your brain engages in a process of imagining potential outcomes.[134]

This ability to mentally test out different scenarios is crucial for effective planning and decision-making. The prefrontal cortex acts as a "simulator," using the cognitive map stored in the hippocampus to test possible actions.[135] This interplay allows us to adapt quickly to new situations and make more informed choices.

Your brain is capable of handling complex, hierarchical decision-making processes.[136] This involves breaking down more significant

[133] How we make complex decisions, by Anne Trafton https://bcs.mit.edu/news/how-we-make-complex-decisions
[134] What's Going On in Our Brains When We Plan? By James Devitt, https://www.nyu.edu/about/news-publications/news/2024/june/what-s-going-on-in-our-brains-when-we-plan-.html
[135] Id.
[136] How we make complex decisions, by Anne Trafton https://bcs.mit.edu/news/how-we-make-complex-decisions

decisions into smaller, more manageable components. For example, when faced with failure or unexpected outcomes for which you are hard-wired in your enchanted forest, your brain performs two key computations:

1. Computing confidence over the outcome of each decision to identify the most likely cause of failure.
2. Making additional attempts to gain more confidence when the cause is not easily discernible.

In this process, your brain flexibly uses episodic memory or information from past experiences, which it recombines in novel ways to imagine future scenarios.[137] Mental simulation is crucial for imagining the many potential outcomes. You are now moving beyond the brain as a prediction machine; you invoke its enhanced awareness and metacognitive skills in creating a picture of the future. This magic places you on the path of calm and, ultimately, to a state of flow, as you will see.

Emotions are crucially important for your choices.[138] The limbic system, including structures like the amygdala and hippocampus, influences your decisions by processing emotions and memories.[139]

Understanding the neuroscience behind decision-making is just the first step. You must shift your mindset to improve your decision-making skills and achieve better results. Here are some strategies based on recent findings:

---

[137] Mullally SL, Maguire EA. Memory, Imagination, and Predicting the Future: A Common Brain Mechanism? Neuroscientist. 2014 Jun;20(3):220-34. doi: 10.1177/1073858413495091. Epub 2013 Jul 11. PMID: 23846418; PMCID: PMC4232337.

[138] Dennison JB, Sazhin D, Smith DV. Decision neuroscience and neuroeconomics: Recent progress and ongoing challenges. Wiley Interdiscip Rev Cogn Sci. 2022 May;13(3):e1589. doi: 10.1002/wcs.1589. Epub 2022 Feb 8. PMID: 35137549; PMCID: PMC9124684.

[139] The Neuroscience of Decision Making, by Sam Dabir, https://uwo.ca/se/thrive/blog/2024/the-neuroscience-of-decision-making.html

1. **Practice mental simulation**: Before making important decisions, take time to imagine different scenarios and their potential outcomes.[140]
2. **Develop a hierarchical approach**: Break down complex decisions into smaller, more manageable components[141]
3. **Consider emotions and social context**: Recognize the influence of emotions and social factors on your decisions. Ask yourself if where you could end up is there where you wanted to be when you started. If the answer is "no," ask yourself "why?"
4. **Cultivate a positive mindset**: Research shows that a positive mindset can enhance coping skills and resilience, leading to better decision-making and health outcomes.[142]
5. **Engage in mindfulness practices**: Regular mindfulness meditation increases gray matter density in brain areas associated with attention, emotional regulation, and self-awareness. Sometimes, you pay a physiological cost for the optimistic strategy of engaging in difficult stressors rather than disengaging and withdrawing.[143] We keep on reverting to conscious awareness as the focal point of transformation.

By understanding and applying these insights, we can move beyond simply focusing on what we want to do or achieve. Your mind is not just a prediction machine. When you use the decision-making processes from your higher center of awareness and are consciously aware, you reflect on

---

[140] What's Going On in Our Brains When We Plan? By James Devitt, June 7th 2024, https://www.nyu.edu/about/news-publications/news/2024/june/what-s-going-on-in-our-brains-when-we-plan-.html

[141] Dennison JB, Sazhin D, Smith DV. Decision neuroscience and neuroeconomics: Recent progress and ongoing challenges. Wiley Interdiscip Rev Cogn Sci. 2022 May;13(3):e1589. doi: 10.1002/wcs.1589. Epub 2022 Feb 8. PMID: 35137549; PMCID: PMC9124684.

[142] Mind Over Matter: How Your Thoughts Shape Your Health, According to Neuroscience, by Dr. Jennifer Ruthensteiner, May 27th, 2023, https://rebootcenter.com/neuroscience-of-mindset/

[143] "This physical cost is reflected in higher cortisol as well as lower cellular immunity. In turn, these costs may affect the course of diseases such as viral infection (e.g., HIV) and some types and stages of cancer for which disruptions in cortisol and cellular immunity are prognostic." Optimism and immunity: do positive thoughts always lead to positive effects? Brain Behav Immun. 2005 May;19(3):195-200. doi: 10.1016/j.bbi.2004.08.003. PMID: 15797306; PMCID: PMC1948078.

your choices and hone the qualities of a visionary world-transformer guided by the future. You can delve deeply into the cognitive processes that shape your decisions and ultimately determine your results. Remember, the key to better results lies in your choices and understanding and optimizing the cognitive processes that drive those decisions.

Exercise For Metacognitive Self-Awareness

1. Confidence Calibration

Think of a recent decision you made. Rate your confidence in that decision on a scale of 1-10, with 1 being not at all confident and 10 being extremely confident. Now, reflect on the actual outcome of that decision. How well did your confidence align with the reality of the situation?

2. Cognitive Strategy Identification

List three strategies you typically use when faced with a challenging decision (e.g., pros and cons list, seeking advice, visualizing outcomes). For each strategy, rate its effectiveness on a scale of 1-5. Which strategy seems most effective, and why?

3. Bias Recognition

Recall a recent situation where you realized you made an error in judgment. What cognitive biases might have influenced your thinking? (e.g., present bias, confirmation bias, availability heuristic, overconfidence)

4. Emotional Impact Assessment

Before making your next important decision, pause and assess your current emotional state. How might your emotions be influencing your thought process? What steps can you take to ensure a more balanced perspective?

5. Adaptive Strategy Application

Think of an upcoming decision you need to make. Based on your reflections from the previous questions, what strategies will you apply to this decision-making process? How will you monitor your thinking and adjust your approach if needed?

WHO ARE YOU REALLY?

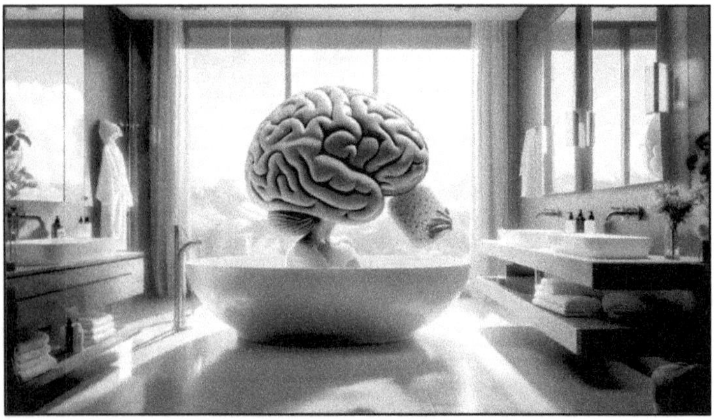

Our fast-paced, technology-driven world is a special version of the enchanted forest. We've become accustomed to instant gratification and quick solutions to our thirst for information and knowledge. This mindset may alter our perception of reality in ways we might not fully appreciate. We need to be cautious about our expectations for instant results.

Our brains are constantly working to make sense of the world around us. Interestingly, what we perceive as reality isn't always an accurate representation of the physical world. Instead, it's a construction based on our expectations, prior experiences, and sensory inputs.[144] Our perceptions are essentially "controlled hallucinations." The brain generates predictions about what it expects to see, hear, or feel and then compares them with sensory input. This process helps us navigate the world efficiently, but it also means that our expectations can influence our perception of reality.

The expectation for instant results can clash with how our brains naturally process information and make decisions. Different parts of our brains compete for control when faced with choices between immediate and delayed rewards. The emotional areas drawn to immediate gratification often conflict with the regions responsible for long-term planning and reasoning.[145] This internal conflict can lead to impulsive decisions and a skewed perception of reality, where we overvalue immediate outcomes and underestimate the importance of long-term consequences.

The intermixing of imagination and perception in our brains presents another challenge to our grasp of reality. Imagined and perceived signals can become subjectively mixed, making distinguishing between real and imagined difficult.[146] [147] It is easy to make decisions based on imaginary information. For example, we can perceive information to be aligned with past experiences, but these experiences, sometimes without our knowledge, are unfavorable to us. Yet, we use them in our predictions. The blurring of lines between reality and imagination is particularly concerning in our current information landscape. With the prevalence of

---

[144] The Neuroscience of Reality, Anil K. Seth, https://www.scientificamerican.com/article/the-neuroscience-of-reality/

[145] Brain takes itself on over immediate vs. delayed gratification, Steve Bradt, https://news.harvard.edu/gazette/story/2004/10/brain-takes-itself-on-over-immediate-vs-delayed-gratification/

[146] Dijkstra N, Fleming SM. Subjective signal strength distinguishes reality from imagination. Nat Commun. 2023 Mar 23;14(1):1627. doi: 10.1038/s41467-023-37322-1. PMID: 36959279; PMCID: PMC10036541.

[147] Dijkstra, N., Fleming, S.M. Subjective signal strength distinguishes reality from imagination. *Nat Commun* **14**, 1627 (2023). https://doi.org/10.1038/s41467-023-37322-1

misinformation and the ease of manipulating digital content, it can be challenging to discern fact from fiction.

To maintain a healthy relationship with reality in this age of instant gratification and information overload, we need to be mindful of how our brains process information. Here are a few strategies:

1. **Practice patience**: Recognize that not everything can or should happen instantly. Cultivate the ability to wait for results and appreciate the process.
2. **Develop critical thinking**: Question your initial perceptions and seek out multiple sources of information before forming conclusions.
3. **Engage in mindfulness**: Regular mindfulness practices can help you become more aware of your thought processes and how they shape your perception of reality.
4. **Limit digital distractions**: Take breaks from constant connectivity to allow your brain time to process information more deeply.
5. **Embrace uncertainty**: Accept that not everything can be known or resolved immediately, and that's okay.

Understand how your brain constructs reality and be aware of the potential pitfalls of our instant-results culture. You can work towards a more balanced and accurate perception of the world around you. It's crucial to remember that true understanding and meaningful progress often require time, patience, and careful consideration.

Have you ever wondered if the person you think you are really **is** "you"? Your self-concept - the beliefs you hold about yourself - is not a fixed entity; it is not set in stone. Instead, it's a fluid and ever-changing representation in your brain. Your brain actively works to maintain a coherent and positive self-image as you encounter new experiences and feedback.[148]

---

[148] A Fluid Self-Concept: How the Brain Maintains Coherence and Positivity across an Interconnected Self-Concept While Incorporating Social Feedback, Jacob J. Elder, Tyler H. Davis and Brent L. Hughes, Journal of Neuroscience 31 May 2023, 43 (22) 4110-4128; https://doi.org/10.1523/JNEUROSCI.1951-22.2023

This process of self-concept-updating involves complex neural mechanisms that help you integrate new information while preserving a sense of consistency. The brain doesn't simply accept all incoming information at face value. Instead, it carefully weighs new feedback against existing beliefs, considering how changes might impact your overall self-image.[149]

Several key brain regions play crucial roles in forming and maintaining your self-concept:

1. The Medial Prefrontal Cortex is a central hub for self-related processing. It's susceptible to information that's important to your self-identity.[150]
2. The ventromedial prefrontal cortex significantly maintains a positive and coherent self-concept.[151]
3. The temporoparietal Junction, particularly its posterior part, is involved in processing social information and distinguishing between self and others.[152]
4. The Angular Gyrus helps manage uncertainty about self-beliefs by considering the relevance of prior feedback.[153]

You can learn your self-concept through your interactions with the world and others. Here's how this learning process unfolds:

---

[149] A Fluid Self-Concept: How the Brain Maintains Coherence and Positivity across an Interconnected Self-Concept While Incorporating Social Feedback, Jacob J. Elder, Tyler H. Davis and Brent L. Hughes Journal of Neuroscience 31 May 2023, 43 (22) 4110-4128; https://doi.org/10.1523/JNEUROSCI.1951-22.2023

[150] Levorsen M, Aoki R, Matsumoto K, Sedikides C, Izuma K. The Self-Concept Is Represented in the Medial Prefrontal Cortex in Terms of Self-Importance. J Neurosci. 2023 May 17;43(20):3675-3686. doi: 10.1523/JNEUROSCI.2178-22.2023. Epub 2023 Apr 7. PMID: 37028931; PMCID: PMC10198449.

[151] A Fluid Self-Concept: How the Brain Maintains Coherence and Positivity across an Interconnected Self-Concept While Incorporating Social Feedback, Jacob J. Elder, Tyler H. Davis and Brent L. Hughes

[152] Nadescha Trudel, Patricia L Lockwood, Matthew FS Rushworth, Marco K Wittmann (2023) Neural activity tracking identity and confidence in social information eLife 12:e71315 https://doi.org/10.7554/eLife.71315

[153] A Fluid Self-Concept: How the Brain Maintains Coherence and Positivity across an Interconnected Self-Concept While Incorporating Social Feedback, Jacob J. Elder, Tyler H. Davis and Brent L. Hughes

1. **Selective Updating**: You learn more quickly from positive than negative feedback about yourself. This bias helps maintain a positive self-image.
2. **Network Dependencies**: Your brain represents traits as part of a network. Traits with more connections (dependencies) in this network are less likely to change in response to feedback.
3. **Back Propagation**: When you receive feedback about one trait, your brain considers how this might affect related traits in your self-concept network.
4. **Retrieval of Past Experiences**: When evaluating yourself, you retrieve information about similar past experiences to inform your current self-views.[154]

Interestingly, your brains seem to process social information differently from non-social information. You tend to be more confident and less changeable in your judgments about social information sources than non-social ones. That's so even though your judgments about social information sources are more prone to the inability to distinguish between what's real and what's not.

You now ask yourself: "If I have a personality trait that my environment has taught me is unfavorable or unwanted, that can seriously and adversely impact my view of who I am? It can override my favorable experiences of other traits I consider genuine?" Yes, that is correct! Especially for a personality trait that is important to you.

You should place so much more emphasis on aligning your world creation to your higher center of awareness so you can shape the world as a visionary creator. You've probably heard that adversity molds character; now you know the reason why. You are probably beginning to realize

[154] A Fluid Self-Concept: How the Brain Maintains Coherence and Positivity across an Interconnected Self-Concept While Incorporating Social Feedback, Jacob J. Elder, Tyler H. Davis and Brent L. Hughes Journal of Neuroscience 31 May 2023, 43 (22) 4110-4128; https://doi.org/10.1523/JNEUROSCI.1951-22.2023

that you have one unchanging, eternal part, and it's not necessarily the many cognitive processes you habitually use to navigate the world daily – especially not those processes you are so convinced will always be there for you! Your consciousness forever watches you, whether you like that or not.

The medial prefrontal cortex plays a key role in representing your self-concept. If a specific identity trait is vital to you, your behaviors in tune with that characteristic will likely be different, more attentive, responsible, or consistent than your behaviors in other, less self-defining roles. The self-importance of a personality trait affects how you seek and remember information about yourself. A dedicated neural system in the brain encodes the self-importance of incoming information, correlated with the importance of possessing a personality trait and the personal significance of autobiographical memories.[155]

The power to be your authentic self is crucial to navigating the enchanted forest. You have probably heard these adages: The weak fall prey to misinformation, and "I love a weak opponent." Some leaders or politicians use these adages to justify unfavorable situations where they do not want change. People with weak self-concepts are easily bogged down to chase illusions in the enchanted forest! That includes people who think their self-concepts are, in reality, strong ones.

Have you ever felt stuck in a cycle of always wanting more but never quite reaching your goals? Many of us operate in a "get" mindset, constantly focused on what we can acquire or achieve yet what we don't appear to reach. This very mindset might be holding you back from true success. There's a more effective way to approach your goals and aspirations. It's all about shifting from a "get" mindset to a "be" mindset.

---

[155] The Self-Concept Is Represented in the Medial Prefrontal Cortex in Terms of Self-Importance
Marie Levorsen, Ryuta Aoki, Kenji Matsumoto, Constantine Sedikides and Keise Izuma
Journal of Neuroscience 17 May 2023, 43 (20) 3675-3686; https://doi.org/10.1523/JNEUROSCI.2178-22.2023

Let's explore why this shift is so powerful and how it can transform your life.

A singular focus on outcomes and acquisitions characterizes the "get" mindset. It's the voice in your head that says, "I want that promotion," "I need more money," or "I have to win this competition." While having goals is essential, this mindset can block your success in several ways:

1. It creates a fixed perspective
2. It leads to constant dissatisfaction
3. It can increase stress and anxiety

When you are solely focused on what you want to get, you often overlook the journey and the personal transformation required on this journey to achieve your goals. You become stuck in a "fixed mindset."[156] This mindset can be entirely at odds with your higher center of awareness towards which you strive. This process can be unconscious.

In contrast, the "be" mindset focuses on who you can become to achieve your goals. This approach is closely related to a "growth mindset."[157] Here's why it's so powerful:

1. **It promotes personal development**: Instead of fixating on the result, you focus on developing the skills and qualities needed to achieve it.
2. **It increases resilience**: When faced with setbacks, you see them as opportunities for growth rather than failures.[158]
3. **It enhances motivation**: Focusing on personal growth makes you more likely to find intrinsic motivation in the process, not just in the end goal.

---

[156] Want to Be More Successful? Neuroscience Shows Embracing a Growth Mindset Actually Changes How Your Brain Functions, https://www.psychologicalscience.org/news/want-to-be-more-successful-neuroscience-shows-embracing-a-growth-mindset-actually-changes-how-your-brain-functions.html

[157] Id.

[158] Your powerful, changeable mindset, https://news.stanford.edu/stories/2021/09/mindsets-clearing-lens-life

4. **It improves brain function**: Neuroscience research shows that embracing a growth mindset changes how your brain functions, making you more open to learning and improvement.[159]

Changing from a "get" to a "be" mindset doesn't happen overnight but is achievable. Here are some strategies to help you make the shift:

1. **Embrace challenges**: Instead of avoiding difficulties, see them as opportunities to grow and learn new skills.
2. **Focus on effort, not just outcomes**: Celebrate your work and see if it is good work that allows you to grow, not just to let you get results.
3. **Use the power of "yet"**: Add "yet" to your statement when faced with a setback. For example, "I haven't mastered this skill... yet."[160]
4. **Practice self-reflection**: Regularly ask yourself, "Who do I need to be to achieve my goals?" rather than just "What do I want to achieve?"
5. **Cultivate a learning orientation**: Approach every situation with curiosity and a desire to learn rather than to prove yourself.

The exciting news about mindsets is that they are completely changeable.[161]

You can shift your perspective and unlock your full potential with conscious effort and practice. By focusing on who you need to be rather than what you want to get, you open yourself up to a world of growth and possibility. You'll find that you achieve your goals more quickly; more importantly, you'll enjoy the journey much more.

---

[159] Want to Be More Successful? Neuroscience Shows Embracing a Growth Mindset Actually Changes How Your Brain Functions, https://www.psychologicalscience.org/news/want-to-be-more-successful-neuroscience-shows-embracing-a-growth-mindset-actually-changes-how-your-brain-functions.html

[160] A Summary of Growth and Fixed Mindsets, by Carol Dweck, https://fs.blog/carol-dweck-mindset/

[161] Your powerful, changeable mindset, September 15, 2021, https://news.stanford.edu/stories/2021/09/mindsets-clearing-lens-life

Exercises to Cultivate Cognitive Flexibility And Heal Rigid Personality Traits

1. Perspective-Shifting

Think of a recent situation where you felt stuck or frustrated. Now, try to view this situation from three different perspectives:

a) How might a close friend see this situation?

b) How would you view this if it happened to someone else?

c) How might you perceive this situation five years from now?

Reflect on how these different viewpoints might change your understanding or emotional response to the situation.

2. Mindfulness Moment

Take 2-3 minutes to practice a brief mindfulness exercise:

- Focus on your breath, noticing the sensation of inhaling and exhaling.
- When thoughts arise, acknowledge them without judgment and gently return your focus to your breath.

This practice has been shown to increase connectivity between brain regions associated with self-awareness and cognitive control, potentially reducing mental rigidity.

3. Creative Problem-Solving

Consider a current challenge in your life. Generate three unconventional or "out-of-the-box" solutions to this problem. They don't need to be practical – the goal is to exercise your ability to think flexibly and creatively.

4. Emotional Labeling

Identify and name three emotions you've experienced today. For each emotion:

a) Describe the physical sensations associated with it.

b) Consider what triggered this emotion.

c) Reflect on how this emotion influenced your thoughts and behaviors.

This practice can help increase emotional granularity and reduce rigid emotional responses.

5. Values Exploration

List three personal values that are important to you. For each value:

a) Describe why it's meaningful to you.

b) Identify a recent situation where you acted in alignment with this value.

c) Consider a way you could express this value more fully in your daily life.

This exercise promotes self-awareness and can help reduce rigidity in self-concept, which is often associated with negative personality traits.

YOU SHINE, YOU ARE AFRAID

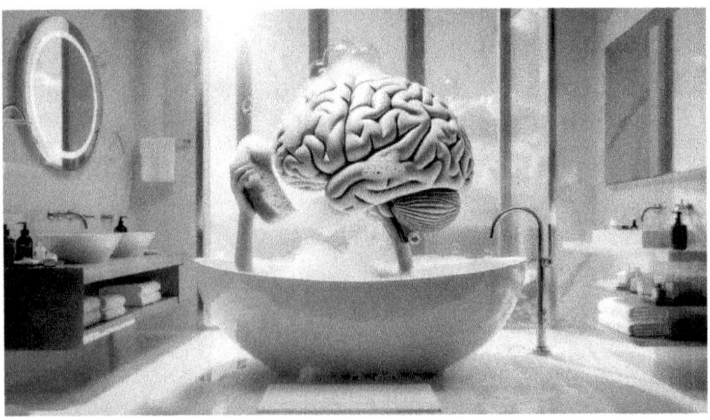

You have figured out by now that there is an eternal, incorruptible, undestroyable part of you that is active 24/7. It's that part from which your awareness and meta-knowledge powers flow, as well as your creativity and your focus. It's the part that embeds you into your origins in the universe. You never have complete access to that part, not because science is not yet sufficiently advanced or because there are skills you still must learn. It is because your perceptions are what you see, and for them to operate healthily in this manner, they require constant input and support from the universe's energy. That energy is always a step ahead of you – a second, a nano-second, or an eternity. The act of seeing requires there is something ahead of your sight.

Even highly attuned people who, for example, accurately know when they will die do not precisely know where they will go after their energy has left their bodies. That is because the energy that supports us, including its transformation, transcends the cognitive faculties we use to bring this energy into this world. "So there is no true transcendental experience?" You will ask. "There is always an element of illusion, or a wrong perception – which can turn into a delusion, or a fixed false belief?" No, there are real transcendental experiences; we have the capacity for those, but they are not permanent. Our transcendental experiences are dependent on their specific purposes. For example, a deceased person cannot send a letter to Earth stating, "My new address is on Street X, on Planet A, and this is the plane, rocket, or spaceship you should take to visit me." While, of course, humans have spoken to their deceased ancestors from the comforts of their homes, and many have assigned great value to these experiences.

More details on these topics are for another book. Let's return to how your eternal part can impact daily life using your sub- or unconsciousness. We have already said that humans have an awareness when they are not conscious. Our minds also operate during slumber, revealing that our subconscious is far more active and alert than we think. Contrary to popular belief, your brain doesn't simply switch off when you drift into dreamland; sleep is not a state of complete unconsciousness. You remain remarkably responsive to the world around you. Sleeping individuals can respond to verbal stimuli by contracting their facial muscles during various sleep stages.[162]

Even when you're deep in slumber, your brain continues to process sensory information from your environment. The human cerebral cortex remains active in response to sounds during sleep, albeit with some key

[162] The lullaby study: re-evaluating consciousness during sleep, https://www.biotechniques.com/neuroscience/the-lullaby-study-re-evaluating-consciousness-during-sleep/

differences compared to the wakeful state.[163] For example, while the brain's feedback signals for interpreting sounds are reduced during sleep, the initial auditory responses remain robust. You may have had the experience of drifting sound while you are asleep. That's also for the additional reason that our cells operate on frequencies.

Your subconscious mind is a tireless worker, constantly processing information and guiding you toward your goals, even when you are unaware. This phenomenon is closely tied to the brain's default mode network, active during mind-wandering and self-reflection.[164] This network is crucial in defining who you are and shaping your aspirations.

Sleep, particularly REM (Rapid Eye Movement) sleep, is vital in memory consolidation and emotional processing.[165] During this stage, your brain "tidies up" recent memories and feelings, helping to solidify learning and solve problems. This is why you might sometimes wake up with a solution to a problem that bothered you the day before!

While you sleep, your brain undergoes a fascinating cleaning process. During REM sleep, the brain essentially "back-flushes" its neural circuits.[166] This process, controlled by the glymphatic system, washes the brain with cerebrospinal fluid, helping to restore cognitive function and prepare you for the next day's mental challenges.

Sleep isn't a uniform state of unconsciousness. Instead, it's more like a mosaic of conscious and seemingly unconscious moments.[167] These

---

[163] Day or night — your brain is always listening, https://new.nsf.gov/news/day-or-night-your-brain-always-listening

[164] How to manifest your future using neuroscience, with James Doty (Ep. 135), https://news.uchicago.edu/manifest-your-future-using-neuroscience-james-doty

[165] REM sleep and the science of dreams: A deep dive into the unconscious mind, https://www.psypost.org/rem-sleep-and-the-science-of-dreams-a-deep-dive-into-the-unconscious-mind/

[166] REM sleep and the science of dreams: A deep dive into the unconscious mind, by Drew Dawson and Madeline Sprajcer, September 24, 2023, https://www.psypost.org/rem-sleep-and-the-science-of-dreams-a-deep-dive-into-the-unconscious-mind/

[167] Türker, B., Musat, E.M., Chabani, E. *et al.* Behavioral and brain responses to verbal stimuli reveal transient periods of cognitive integration of the external world during sleep. *Nat Neurosci* **26**, 1981–1993 (2023). https://doi.org/10.1038/s41593-023-01449-7

"windows of consciousness" during sleep might explain why some people report being able to solve problems or gain insights while dreaming. So, how can we harness sleep to heighten our awareness?

Enhancing awareness during sleep, also known as lucid dreaming, can be achieved through various techniques and practices. Here are two effective methods to work on increasing your awareness while sleeping:

The Mnemonic Induction of Lucid Dreams (MILD) technique is one of the most effective methods for inducing lucid dreams. Here's how to practice it:

1. Wake up after 5-6 hours of sleep
2. Recall a recent dream
3. Identify a "dreamsign" - something unusual that only occurs in dreams
4. Repeat the phrase: "Next time I'm dreaming, I will remember I'm dreaming."
5. Visualize yourself becoming lucid in the dream
6. Fall back asleep while focusing on this intention.[168]

The Wake Back to Bed (WBTB) method involves waking up during the night and then returning to sleep with the intention of lucid dreaming.

1. Set an alarm for 5 hours after your bedtime
2. When the alarm goes off, stay awake for 30 minutes
3. Engage in a quiet activity like reading about lucid dreaming or any reading or thinking that you associate with mindfulness
4. Return to sleep, focusing on your intention to become lucid.[169]

---

[168] How to Lucid Dream: Expert Tips and Tricks, by Lucy Bryan and Dr. Abhinav Singh, September 20, 2024, https://www.sleepfoundation.org/dreams/lucid-dreams

[169] 5 Lucid Dreaming Techniques to Try, Karin Gepp, PsyD, March 22, 2023, https://www.healthline.com/health/healthy-sleep/how-to-lucid-dream

Have you been enhancing your subconscious, but you have trouble falling asleep? Here is a technique that I find especially useful to drift to sleep calmly:

1. Bring to mind a mantra that gave your life meaning; it can be a mantra you discovered as a child or that you located during your work on your subconscious
2. Focus on the intention of your mantra and continue to repeat your mantra
3. Calmly breath yourself into sleep while you continue to repeat your mantra

You may notice you don't enter sleep as you know it but a heightened state of calm awareness that becomes your sleep.

As you practice these techniques consistently, you will become better and better at them. You will no longer experience your 'getting up' in the morning as an unwelcomed disturbance.

You will gain many benefits by working on your subconscious. Your subconscious mind plays a crucial role in goal selection and achievement. It's often making decisions before you are aware of them.[170] By the time you consciously pursue a goal, your subconscious has already been hard at work, influencing your choices. But your subconscious isn't just randomly picking goals out of thin air. It's deeply influenced by something even more fundamental - your identity.

Think of your identity as the operating system for your subconscious mind. It's the set of beliefs, values, and self-perceptions that define who you think you are. This identity acts as a filter, determining which goals align with your self-image and which don't.[171] For example, if you see

[170] New Insights into the Neuroscience Behind Conscious Awareness of Choice, https://www.caltech.edu/about/news/new-insights-into-the-neuroscience-behind-conscious-awareness-of-choice

[171] BLUEPRINTS FOR SUCCESS: NEUROSCIENTIFIC PRINCIPLES BEHIND EFFECTIVE GOAL SETTING, https://mindlabneuroscience.com/goal-setting/

yourself as a health-conscious person, your subconscious is more likely to choose and pursue goals related to fitness and nutrition. Conversely, if you identify as someone who struggles with self-discipline, your subconscious might sabotage efforts to stick to a strict routine – even if your struggle with self-discipline is not always clear to you.

Once your subconscious has selected a goal that aligns with your identity, it becomes a relentless achiever. Your brain's reticular activating system kicks into high gear, filtering information and opportunities that can help you reach your goal.[172] It's like having a personal assistant constantly looking for ways to make your goals a reality. But here's the catch: this goal-achieving machine works just as hard for goals that might not serve you well. If you have a deeply ingrained belief that it's better for you to wait, or to practice avoidance, your subconscious will work tirelessly to find evidence to support that belief, even if it's not in your best interest.[173]

So, how can you use this knowledge to your advantage? The key lies in shaping your identity to align with the goals you want to achieve. Here are a few strategies:

1. **Reframe your identity**: Instead of saying, "I want to lose weight," try "I am a healthy person who takes care of my body."
2. **Visualize success**: Regularly imagine yourself achieving your goals. This helps program your subconscious to seek out opportunities for success.[174]
3. **Practice mindfulness**: Knowing your thoughts and beliefs can help you identify and change limiting self-perceptions.[175]

---

[172] The Reticular Activating System: How Goal-Setting and Manifesting Work in the Brain, https://anthonyvlombardo.com/goal-setting-brain/

[173] Identity Works Because It Creates A Need, https://www.selfimprovementdailytips.com/podcast/identity-works-because-it-creates-a-need

[174] BLUEPRINTS FOR SUCCESS: NEUROSCIENTIFIC PRINCIPLES BEHIND EFFECTIVE GOAL SETTING, https://mindlabneuroscience.com/goal-setting/

[175] Unconscious Mind: How Our Beliefs and Experiences Shape Our Lives, by Albert Wong, Ph.D., Mar 04, 2023, https://www.somatopia.com/blog/unconscious-mind-techniques

4. **Set identity-based goals**: Focus on becoming the person who would achieve your desired outcome rather than just on the outcome itself.

Remember, your mind is a potent tool. By understanding how your subconscious and identity work together, you can harness this power to achieve the goals that genuinely matter to you. So reflect on how you may want to BE instead of chasing after goals, and let your goal-achieving machine trust YOU to find its way.

Have you ever wondered about the depths of who you are? The journey of self-mastery is all about peeling back the layers of your consciousness and getting to know your true essence. For a long time, there's been a debate about whether the "self" is authentic or just another illusion. But guess what? Recent neuroscience suggests that the self is real – just not how we might think.

Your self is not something you can hold in your hand but rather an "informational entity" that emerges from the complex processes in our brains. Think of it like this: your brain is constantly creating a model of the world around you, and part of that model includes you! This self-modeling process involves brain networks like the cortical midline structures and the default mode network.[176] These networks light up when we self-reflect, daydream, or think about the future.

Now, let's talk about self-mastery. It's not just a fancy term – it's a lifelong personal growth and development process. At its core, self-mastery is about gaining control over your thoughts, emotions, and actions. It's like becoming the captain of your ship, navigating through the uncertain, sometimes stormy seas of the enchanted forest. To embark on this journey, you need to develop self-awareness and learn to regulate your thoughts and emotions

[176] Actually, neuroscience suggests "the self" is real, https://bigthink.com/the-well/actually-neuroscience-suggests-self-real/

By doing so, you're not just improving yourself – you're enhancing your ability to handle stress, make better decisions, and build stronger relationships.[177]

Here's where it gets exciting. Your conscious experience plays a crucial role in building your sense of self.[178] It's not just about what you think you know about yourself but about how you experience these thoughts, feelings, and actions. Imagine your consciousness as a vast, fluid universe. Self-mastery is like learning to dive deeper and deeper into this universe of you, exploring its depths and discovering hidden treasures. As you dive, you might encounter:

- Cognitive self-consciousness: Your awareness of your thoughts and mental processes
- Bodily self-consciousness: Your sense of your physical self and its boundaries
- Spatial self-consciousness: Your awareness of where you are in relation to your environment.[179]

As you continue your journey of self-mastery and are no longer the prey of the enchanted forest, you'll start to get glimpses of your true essence. This isn't some mystical concept – it's grounded in neuroscience. Your essence is the core part that emerges from all these complex brain processes. Remember, your self isn't a fixed entity. It's a dynamic process that's constantly evolving. Every time you are mindfully present in the moment, reflect on your abilities, or make a new decision challenging yourself with new experiences, you're reinforcing and modifying your sense of self.[180] Self-mastery isn't about reaching a final destination. Keep

---

[177] Self-Mastery Explained, https://www.warriors.co.za/articles/Self-Mastery-Explained

[178] Marchetti G (2024) The self and conscious experience. *Front. Psychol.* 15:1340943. doi: 10.3389/fpsyg.2024.1340943

[179] Marchetti G (2024) The self and conscious experience. *Front. Psychol.* 15:1340943. doi: 10.3389/fpsyg.2024.1340943

[180] Self-mastery explained, by Rudi Viljoen, July 3, 2024, https://www.warriors.co.za/articles/Self-Mastery-Explained

exploring, questioning, and diving deeper into your consciousness's fascinating universe.

Have you had a moment where you felt like you broke free from your usual patterns and connected with something greater? Let's explore what happens in your brain during these profound moments of self-transcendence. When you pierce through your conditioning and connect with something beyond yourself, you tap into complex neural networks in our brains. The brain regions involved in self-awareness and consciousness give clues about what might happen during these transformative experiences.

One key player in self-awareness is the Default Mode Network (DMN), a group of interconnected brain regions that become active when you are at rest, engaged in self-reflection, or not focused on the outside world.[181] This network, which includes the medial prefrontal cortex or mPFC, is involved in autobiographical memory and imagining the future. This network allows you to step back from your immediate experiences and reflect on your identity in a broader context. It's like your brain's built-in meditation system constantly works to maintain and update your sense of self. During moments of self-transcendence, activity in the DMN may shift, allowing you to step outside your usual self-referential thinking patterns temporarily. This could explain the expanded awareness many people report during these experiences.

Another important neural system is the Salience Network, which includes the insula and anterior cingulate cortex.[182] This network helps you identify what's important or relevant in your environment. When you have a transcendent experience, the Salience Network might highlight novel or meaningful aspects of your consciousness that you

---

[181] The Neuroscience Behind Self-Awareness: Understanding the Brain's Role in Self-Perception, https://www.perfectequilibrium.co/insights/the-neuroscience-behind-self-awareness-understanding-the-brains-role-in-self-perception

[182] Overgaard, M., Preston, C. & Aspell, J. The self, its body and its brain. *Sci Rep* **13**, 12761 (2023). https://doi.org/10.1038/s41598-023-39959-w

don't typically notice. Self-awareness integrates sensory, emotional, and cognitive information across various brain networks.[183] A transcendent experience may temporarily alter this integration process, allowing new perspectives and insights to emerge. The brain's ability to form new connections and reorganize itself, known as neural plasticity, plays a crucial role in our breakthroughs. When you have a moment of insight or expanded awareness, new neural pathways are likely to be formed or strengthened.[184]

At the heart of these experiences is the enigma of consciousness itself. The "default ascending arousal network" (DAAN) in the brain integrates wakefulness and self-awareness and could be called a consciousness network.[185] [186] This network connects various brain regions, including the brainstem and higher cognitive areas, providing a neuroanatomical foundation for conscious experience.

Interestingly, self-awareness isn't confined to specific brain areas but emerges from diffuse interactions among brain networks. Four fascinating factors that play prominently in this emergence are dopamine or the feel-good hormone; oxygen; energy in its proper physical action and form, which can be the resting or floating energy place that is the purpose of Yoga; and energy in its proper conscious or mental action, or mindfulness meditation.[187] [188] This emerging, distributed nature of

---

[183] Overgaard, M., Preston, C. & Aspell, J. The self, its body and its brain. *Sci Rep* **13**, 12761 (2023). https://doi.org/10.1038/s41598-023-39959-w

[184] Mapping human consciousness: A breakthrough study, Eric W. Dolan, https://www.psypost.org/mapping-human-consciousness-a-breakthrough-study/#google_vignette

[185] Mapping human consciousness: A breakthrough study, Eric W. Dolan, https://www.psypost.org/mapping-human-consciousness-a-breakthrough-study/#google_vignette

[186] Multimodal MRI reveals brainstem connections that sustain wakefulness in human consciousness.*Sci. Transl. Med.***16**,eadj4303(2024).DOI:10.1126/scitranslmed.adj4303

[187] Self-Awareness: The Brain Science Behind This Cognitive State & What New Research Says, https://www.endominance.com/blog/2021/09/03/self-awareness-the-brain-science-behind-this-cognitive-state-what-new-research-says/

[188] H.C. Lou, J.P. Changeux, A. Rosenstand, Towards a cognitive neuroscience of self-awareness, Neuroscience & Biobehavioral Reviews, Volume 83, 2017, Pages 765-773, ISSN 0149-7634, https://doi.org/10.1016/j.neubiorev.2016.04.004.

consciousness might explain why transcendent experiences can feel so all-encompassing and difficult to localize.

Connecting with something beyond ourselves, even for a split second, can profoundly affect our sense of self and well-being. These experiences often involve a shift in perspective, allowing us to see beyond our usual limitations. This expanded viewpoint can lead to increased creativity and problem-solving abilities. Expanded self-awareness is closely linked to emotional intelligence and emotion regulation.[189] Moments of transcendence may enhance your ability to understand and manage your emotions, leading to feelings of peace, clarity, or insight.

Expanded self-awareness can guide your sense of self. At the heart of our self-awareness network lies a remarkable brain region called the medial prefrontal cortex (mPFC). This area plays a crucial role in how you perceive and understand yourself. It's the brain's personal identity center, constantly processing information about who you are and what matters to you. The mPFC is particularly active when you think about essential things to your self-identity. Your sense of self isn't just a vague feeling – it's a concrete neural representation in your brain.

The mPFC doesn't just light up when you think about any old thing related to you. It's tuned explicitly to aspects of yourself that you consider essential.[190] This means that how you value different parts of your identity directly impacts your brain activity. So, when you feel like there's an untapped potential within you, your brain might be trying to tell you something important about who you are.

---

[189] The Neuroscience Behind Self-Awareness: Understanding the Brain's Role in Self-Perception, https://www.perfectequilibrium.co/insights/the-neuroscience-behind-self-awareness-understanding-the-brains-role-in-self-perception

[190] Levorsen M, Aoki R, Matsumoto K, Sedikides C, Izuma K. The Self-Concept Is Represented in the Medial Prefrontal Cortex in Terms of Self-Importance. J Neurosci. 2023 May 17;43(20):3675-3686. doi: 10.1523/JNEUROSCI.2178-22.2023. Epub 2023 Apr 7. PMID: 37028931; PMCID: PMC10198449.

But while your brain has this incredible capacity for self-awareness, you don't develop your sense of self in isolation. How you perceive and interact with your environment plays a massive role in shaping how you see yourself. These external factors can sometimes overshadow your internal sense of self, leading you to adopt beliefs about yourself that might not truly reflect your core identity. That's so, primarily if you pursue rigid thought patterns, impulsive solutions, quick satisfactions, and cozy corners, to name a few; you now know how easy that can be! There is, in other words, nothing more valuable you can do for yourself than train and enable your expanded self-awareness to guide your sense of self.

So, what can you do if you feel like you've lost touch with your authentic self? Here are a few science-backed suggestions:

1. **Practice mindfulness**: Mindfulness meditation has been shown to enhance activity in brain regions associated with self-awareness.
2. **Engage in self-reflection**: Take time to journal or think deeply about your values, goals, and what truly matters to you.
3. **Challenge limiting beliefs**: Remember that others may have influenced your beliefs about yourself. Question whether these beliefs truly reflect your authentic self.
4. **Explore new experiences**: Trying new things can help you discover aspects of yourself you may have overlooked.
5. **Seek supportive relationships**: Surround yourself with people who encourage you to be authentic.

Your brain has an incredible capacity for self-awareness and personal growth. The "you" you seek isn't some distant, unattainable ideal – it's already there, waiting to be recognized and nurtured. By understanding the neuroscience of self-awareness, you can learn to tune into your authentic self more effectively. So next time you feel that spark of potential within you, know it's not just your imagination – it's your brain telling you about the amazing person you indeed are.

Your brain processes information hundreds of millions of times faster than chemical processes alone. A quantum effect called superradiance in your neuron networks occurs on an incredibly fast timescale of less than a picosecond. This effect offers protection against degenerative disease and ultra-fast transmission of quantum signals in the brain.[191] This quantum leap in information processing speed could explain the brain's ability to perform complex computations and generate conscious experiences with remarkable efficiency.

The Nested Observer Windows (NOW) Model proposes a hierarchical structure of consciousness where information is processed across multiple spatiotemporal scales in the brain.[192] This model suggests that unified consciousness exists at the apex of a vast nested hierarchy, integrating information from various levels of neural activity. Quantum integration might explain how the brain resolves conflicting thoughts and generates a coherent sense of self.

Tryptophan, an essential amino acid found in various biological structures, including neurons, has been identified as a key player in quantum-level brain processes. When arranged in large, symmetrical networks within neural structures, tryptophan molecules exhibit a remarkable quantum property known as "superradiance."[193] This phenomenon allows tryptophan networks to absorb and re-emit light particles (photons) more efficiently than individual molecules.[194]

---

[191] Quantum biology's new frontier: Tryptophan networks and brain disease defense, April 29, 2024, https://www.news-medical.net/news/20240429/Quantum-biologys-new-frontier-Tryptophan-networks-and-brain-disease-defense.aspx

[192] Justin Riddle, Jonathan W Schooler, Hierarchical consciousness: the Nested Observer Windows model, Neuroscience of Consciousness, Volume 2024, Issue 1, 2024, niae010, https://doi.org/10.1093/nc/niae010

[193] Researchers Discover Protective Quantum Effect in the Brain, April 29, 2024, https://scienceblog.com/544062/researchers-discover-protective-quantum-effect-in-the-brain/

[194] Quantum optical phenomenon in the brain challenges conventional view of amyloid in Alzheimer's, August 25, 2024, https://www.eurekalert.org/news-releases/1055890

Tryptophan networks can efficiently absorb damaging UV light and re-emit it at safer energy levels, potentially protecting the brain from oxidative stress associated with conditions like Alzheimer's. These networks may function as quantum fiber optics, enabling the brain to process information hundreds of millions of times faster than traditional chemical processes alone.[195] [196]

Large-scale quantum coherence in tryptophan mega-networks could underlie the brain's ability to integrate information from various regions, creating a unified conscious experience. The collective amplification of quantum phenomena in neural structures may give rise to higher-order, emergent properties such as self-awareness and unified consciousness. Tryptophan networks exhibit long-range collective quantum coherence, potentially facilitating information integration across distant brain regions and contributing to a cohesive sense of self.[197] An additional reason why your emerging, expanded self-awareness should guide your sense of self!

Narration and building worlds by means of narration, which we humans call "creative fiction," may be the easiest way to take advantage of our quantum abilities. Narration employs specific cognitive mechanisms that can be highly beneficial to you. Engaging with fictional worlds can play a crucial role in expanding our mental horizons. Imaginary worlds may have evolutionary advantages, encouraging spatial exploration and grabbing our attention through exaggerated details. Cognitive neuroscience has revealed the importance of perspective-taking in broadening our understanding of reality. Engaging in activities like role-playing or immersing ourselves in stories activates brain regions

---

[195] Brain's Quantum Fiber Optics May Combat Alzheimer's, April 30, 2024, https://quantumzeitgeist.com/brains-quantum-fiber-optics-may-combat-alzheimers/

[196] Researchers Discover Protective Quantum Effect in the Brain, April 29, 2024, https://scienceblog.com/544062/researchers-discover-protective-quantum-effect-in-the-brain/

[197] Long-range Collective Quantum Coherence in Tryptophan Mega-Networks of Biological Architectures, https://spacefed.com/biology/long-range-collective-quantum-coherence-in-tryptophan-mega-networks-of-biological-architectures/

associated with complex cognitive processes. This neural activity helps us develop a more nuanced and flexible worldview.

Here are some practical steps to create your varied, expansive consciousness:

1. Engage with diverse perspectives: Seek out information and viewpoints that challenge your existing beliefs.
2. Practice mindfulness: Pay attention to your thoughts and assumptions without judgment.
3. Explore fictional worlds: Read books, watch movies, or play games that transport you to different realities.
4. Reflect on your experiences: Take time to question why you interpret events the way you do.
5. Embrace uncertainty: Recognize that your current understanding of reality may be limited or flawed.

The human mind is a remarkable instrument, capable of creating vivid experiences and shaping our perception of reality. However, our perception of the world as our brains actively construct our reality is not as straightforward as we might think, and this is where narration can lend us an invaluably helping hand. As we discussed, rather than passively receiving sensory information, our brains constantly generate predictions about the world around us. This process has its roots in the ideas of 19th-century physicist Hermann von Helmholtz, who proposed that perception is a process of unconscious inference.

What you perceive is not a direct representation of reality but rather a "controlled hallucination."[198] Your brain creates a model of the world based on sensory inputs and expectations. When these predictions match incoming sensory data, you perceive a stable reality. However, when there's a mismatch, your brain updates its models, which should lead to new perceptions or insights. But it's not as easy.

[198] The Neuroscience of Reality, https://www.scientificamerican.com/article/the-neuroscience-of-reality/

Most importantly, your brain encounters a mismatch more often than not. You could say you are wired to encounter mismatches. Unconscious inferences, by definition, involve us with uncertainty and fear. You guessed correctly: Narration is what the enchanted forest is made of – for us! And as we will now see, fear is the primary indicator that we are preparing to break through this uncertainty.

Your perceptions, beliefs, and expectations form the boundaries of your mental construct. You often don't realize these limitations until you encounter something that challenges your existing mental models, and fear indicates that you have made this encounter. When you discover information or experiences that don't fit your existing mental models – this, again, can be most of the time - it triggers fear or anxiety. This emotional response might be seen as a "shock," signaling that you have reached what appears to be the edge of your mental abilities.[199]

To discover the infinite reality beyond your mind, you need to be willing to challenge your existing mental models. This process involves:

1. **Recognizing your biases**: Understanding that prior experiences and expectations influence your perceptions.
2. **Embracing uncertainty**: Being open to new information, even when it challenges your existing beliefs.
3. **Cultivating curiosity**: Actively seeking out diverse experiences and perspectives to expand your mental models.

It's only by harnessing your quantum self to integrate your self-concept so as to navigate uncertainty that you can successfully pave your way through the realm of fear with an expansive consciousness. The realm of fear is extraordinarily pervasive; it makes itself ever present to us by the slightest rustle in the leaves. Merely expecting to see a specific image can

[199] Wang, J., E, M., Wu, Q. *et al.* Influence of Perceptual and Conceptual Information on Fear Generalization: A Behavioral and Event-Related Potential Study. *Cogn Affect Behav Neurosci* **21**, 1054–1065 (2021). https://doi.org/10.3758/s13415-021-00912-x

activate a neural representation of that image in the deep layers of the early visual cortex, even when nothing is presented to the eyes.[200] In addition, perceptual cues of fear often elicit stronger fear responses than conceptual ones.[201] We are amazingly well covered in the face of experiencing fear.

We might sometimes be trapped in patterns of thinking we've created ourselves. Even if our mental patterns are causing us distress, we often cling to them because they're familiar. This is partly due to the brain's preference for predictability, which activates reward centers and provides security.[202] Stepping outside our mental comfort zone triggers the brain's fear response. The amygdala, a key player in processing emotions, becomes hyperactive when faced with uncertainty or potential threats.[203] This can overwhelm the prospect of change, even when our current situation is less than ideal, and we would want a change. Especially then.

Our brain's defensive circuits are continuously engaged when we're constantly in a state of heightened alertness. Circuits of anxiety form in response to uncertainty or potential threats.[204] This can lead to a distorted perception of reality, where we mistake our fear responses for everyday life experiences.[205] Prolonged states of fear and anxiety can have

---

[200] Great Expectations: How Our Prior Experiences Shape Our Reality, https://www.cogneurosociety.org/great-expectations-how-our-prior-experiences-shape-our-reality/

[201] Wang, J., E, M., Wu, Q. *et al.* Influence of Perceptual and Conceptual Information on Fear Generalization: A Behavioral and Event-Related Potential Study. *Cogn Affect Behav Neurosci* **21**, 1054–1065 (2021). https://doi.org/10.3758/s13415-021-00912-x

[202] Berns GS, McClure SM, Pagnoni G, Montague PR. Predictability modulates human brain response to reward. J Neurosci. 2001 Apr 15;21(8):2793-8. doi: 10.1523/JNEUROSCI.21-08-02793.2001. PMID: 11306631; PMCID: PMC6762527.

[203] LeDoux, J. E., & Pine, D. S. (2016). Using Neuroscience to Help Understand Fear and Anxiety: A Two-System Framework. *American Journal of Psychiatry, 173*(11), 1083–1093. https://doi.org/10.1176/appi.ajp.2016.16030353

[204] Using Neuroscience to Help Understand Fear and Anxiety: A Two-System Framework, Joseph E. LeDoux, Ph.D., and Daniel S. Pine, M.D., American Journal of Psychiatry, Volume 173, Number 11, https://doi.org/10.1176/appi.ajp.2016.16030353

[205] LeDoux, J. E., & Pine, D. S. (2016). Using Neuroscience to Help Understand Fear and Anxiety: A Two-System Framework. *American Journal of Psychiatry, 173*(11), 1083–1093. https://doi.org/10.1176/appi.ajp.2016.16030353 ; Taschereau-Dumouchel, V., Michel, M., Lau,

significant effects on our brain's ability to function optimally. Executive functions like attention, memory, and problem-solving can be impaired. Emotional regulation becomes more challenging. Our ability to process and interpret social cues may be affected.

Embracing uncertainty with self-compassion can help rewire neural pathways associated with fear and anxiety. Developing self-compassion can counteract the adverse effects of self-criticism and shame, which often reinforce our mental prisons. Self-compassion activates different neural networks associated with positive emotions and self-soothing.[206]

When you think of fear, you often imagine it as a signal to retreat or avoid danger. Instead, fear can be a powerful motivator for personal growth and achievement. Rather than seeing fear as a sign to run away, you can reframe it as an indicator to move forward. Let's explore how this perspective shift can transform your relationship with fear and unlock your potential.

At its core, fear is a complex emotional response that involves several brain regions working in concert. The amygdala, often called the brain's "fear center," is crucial in processing emotional stimuli. Interestingly, the neurochemical reactions triggered by fear are strikingly similar to those associated with excitement. Both fear and excitement activate the sympathetic nervous system, leading to increased heart rate, elevated blood pressure, heightened sensory awareness, and release of stress hormones like cortisol and adrenaline. This similarity in physiological responses provides a unique opportunity. By consciously reframing your interpretation of these bodily sensations, you can shift your experience from fear to excitement.

H. *et al.* Putting the "mental" back in "mental disorders": a perspective from research on fear and anxiety. *Mol Psychiatry* **27**, 1322–1330 (2022). https://doi.org/10.1038/s41380-021-01395-5

[206] Maryam Sajadian, Seyed Jalal Younesi, Parvin Jafari, Manouchehr Azkhosh, Razieh Bidhendi Yarandi, Mohammadreza Kordbagheri, Shame, fear of compassion, self-criticism, and self-reassurance mediate the effect of early life events on emotional disorders among male prisoners: A structural equation modeling analysis, Acta Psychologica, Volume 242, 2024, 104116, ISSN 0001-6918, https://doi.org/10.1016/j.actpsy.2023.104116.

Cognitive reappraisal is central to understanding how to transform fear into a motivational force. This process involves consciously changing your interpretation of a situation, which can alter your emotional experience. When faced with a fear-inducing situation, you can pause and reassess. Instead of viewing the physical sensations as signs of danger, you can interpret them as indicators of readiness and anticipation. This shift in perspective can turn a potentially paralyzing experience into an energizing one.

Embracing fear as a catalyst for growth means embracing a growth mindset. You can develop your skills and abilities with effort and practice; they are not fixed traits. When you engage in challenging experiences, even those that initially provoke fear, you actively rewire your brain for resilience and adaptability.[207]

Fear can be a powerful motivator when harnessed correctly. Maybe you realized that, on a profound level, you fear precisely those actions that could benefit you. Think about it: What do you fear most from within the treacherous safety of the enchanted forest? The blinding light of day that will leave none of those comforting shadows! That's right; how afraid are you of the clear awareness that all you have ever held dear is a lie?

Fear, when employed correctly, can cut through present bias, encouraging you to take actions that benefit your future self; fear can enhance focus and alertness, helping you channel your energy into the task at hand; fear can trigger your loss aversion bias, motivating you to work harder to maintain what is to your benefit so that you can evolve. It's crucial to strike a balance. While fear can be motivating in the short term, relying solely on fear-based motivation over the long term can lead to burnout and anxiety.[208]

---

[207] The Science of "Doing It Scared": How Fear and Excitement Can Move You Forward, July 10, 2024, https://www.lumiacoaching.com/blog/how-fear-and-excitement-can-move-you-forward-as-a-coach
[208] Fear As a Motivator: The Benefits and Caveats, February 3, 2023, Alisha Verly Jensen

When your "thinking" brain provides feedback to your "emotional" brain that you are in the safe space of resting energy, you can quickly shift your experience from fear to excitement or enjoyment. Yoga aficionados know: You are afraid that you can't hold a challenging pose until you enter that spot of resting energy. That's when you no longer fear the challenge – even if the pose is challenging!

Your sense of control plays a vital role in this process. When you recognize what is and isn't a real threat and feel confident in your ability to handle the situation, you are more likely to experience fear as a positive, motivating force.[209] The next time you feel fear rising, remember: it might just be your brain's way of telling you that you're on the brink of an exciting opportunity for growth and achievement.

What you often mistake for "life itself" may be your brain's overactive protection mechanisms. With patience and practice, you can learn to distinguish between genuine threats and the echoes of your fears, opening yourself up to a richer, more fulfilling life experience.

Have you ever wondered why certain events trigger negative thoughts and emotions, especially regarding love and relationships? At the core of this issue lies the intricate workings of our brain's limbic system. This system, which includes the amygdala, hippocampus, and prefrontal cortex, plays a crucial role in processing emotions and memories.

When you practice self-love, on the other hand, something remarkable happens in your brain:

1. The prefrontal cortex, responsible for self-awareness and self-control, becomes more active.
2. The amygdala, which processes negative emotions like fear and anxiety, shows decreased activity.

[209] What Happens in the Brain When We Feel Fear, October 27, 2017, Arash Javanbakht and Linda Saab https://www.smithsonianmag.com/science-nature/what-happens-brain-feel-fear-180966992/

3. Dopamine, the "feel-good" neurotransmitter, is released, reinforcing positive behaviors.[210]

This neurological dance creates a positive feedback loop, encouraging you to continue engaging in self-love activities and improving your overall emotional well-being. On the flip side, when you don't love yourself enough, you often fall into the trap of self-criticism. This negative self-talk can have profound effects on your brain and behavior:

1. It increases activity in the amygdala while decreasing activity in the prefrontal cortex, leading to emotional dysregulation.
2. Stress hormones like cortisol are released, negatively impacting physical and emotional health.[211]
3. You tend to suppress your emotions and conceal your thoughts and feelings, damaging your social relationships.

When you struggle with self-love, it can significantly affect your ability to form and maintain loving relationships. Self-critical individuals often mute their emotional expressions, particularly positive ones. This can make it difficult for others to connect with them emotionally. The tendency to self-concealment hides personal information perceived as negative and can create barriers in relationships, preventing deep, meaningful connections.[212] Your self-doubt can become a negative self-fulfilling prophecy, hindering personal growth and fulfillment in relationships.[213]

On the other hand, reflecting on personal core values activates brain regions associated with self-processing and positive valuation, such as the

---

[210] Self-Love and the Neuroscience Behind It, by Dennis Relojo-Howell, 19 February 2023, https://www.psychreg.org/self-love-neuroscience-behind-it/

[211] Id.

[212] New Research Sheds Light on How Self-Criticism Damages Social Relationships, https://portlandpsychotherapy.com/2023/10/new-research-sheds-light-on-how-self-criticism-damages-social-relationships/

[213] Self-Criticism: What it is And How it is Harmful, 12 February 2024, https://mitsu.care/blog/what-is-self-criticism/

medial prefrontal cortex and ventral striatum.[214] Sharing happiness, excitement, and affection can significantly improve relationship development and maintenance.[215] Treating yourself with the same kindness and understanding you would offer a friend can help balance out self-critical thoughts. Measure your progress against your own values and expectations, not against those of others! This can reduce self-criticism and boost self-worth.[216]

In the shadowy corners of your mind, fears often lurk unnoticed, silently shaping your thoughts and behaviors. These hidden fears can profoundly influence your life, often without your conscious awareness. Your brain is remarkably adept at processing fear, a crucial survival mechanism that has evolved over millennia. This system can work against you, especially when fear responses become generalized or exaggerated once your brain's "fear switch" is turned on. Acute stress can cause specific neurons to change their chemical signals, switching from producing excitatory glutamate to inhibitory GABA. This switch in the brainstem's dorsal raphe area appears to be a key factor in generalizing fear responses.[217]

When you experience a traumatic event, your brain doesn't just store that specific memory. Instead, it often generalizes the fear, applying it to a broader range of situations. For instance, if a dog bites you, you might develop a fear not just of that particular dog or of all dogs but also of places associated with dogs or smells that may indicate a dog.

---

[214] Cascio CN, O'Donnell MB, Tinney FJ, Lieberman MD, Taylor SE, Strecher VJ, Falk EB. Self-affirmation activates brain systems associated with self-related processing and reward and is reinforced by future orientation. Soc Cogn Affect Neurosci. 2016 Apr;11(4):621-9. doi: 10.1093/scan/nsv136. Epub 2015 Nov 5. PMID: 26541373; PMCID: PMC4814782.

[215] New Research Sheds Light on How Self-Criticism Damages Social Relationships, https://portlandpsychotherapy.com/2023/10/new-research-sheds-light-on-how-self-criticism-damages-social-relationships/

[216] Self-Criticism: What it is And How it is Harmful, 12 February 2024, https://mitsu.care/blog/what-is-self-criticism/

[217] Fear Switch in the Brain May Point to Target for Treating Anxiety Disorders Including PTSD, by Dr. Monica M. Bertagnolli, April 4th, 2024, https://directorsblog.nih.gov/2024/04/04/fear-switch-in-the-brain-may-point-to-target-for-treating-anxiety-disorders-including-ptsd/

This generalization of fear can act like an invisible puppet master, pulling the strings of your behavior without your conscious awareness. It's as if your brain, in its zealous attempt to protect you, casts a wide net of caution that can entangle unrelated aspects of your life. These generalized fears infiltrate your existing neural networks. Fear-related brain activity patterns can spread to seemingly unrelated categories of information.[218] A traumatic experience can lead to a cascade of fears that may seem irrational on the surface. The fear switch persists for a significant period after the stressful event.

Glucocorticoid receptors are key to the stress response and enhance the consolidation of fear memories.[219] Stressed individuals with high levels of fear or anxiety tend to exhibit more rigid thinking patterns.[220] Psychological rigidity exhibits strong positive associations with negative processes, suggesting that inflexible thinking is closely tied to negative emotions and thoughts.[221] Psychological rigidity, or cognitive inflexibility, tends to persist in particular thought patterns or behaviors, even when they're no longer effective or beneficial. This rigidity can manifest in various aspects of our lives, from approaching problem-solving to interacting with others.

You often fail to see alternative perspectives or solutions when stuck in rigid thinking patterns. This inflexibility can lead you to:

1. Overlook potential solutions to problems;
2. Miss out on new experiences;
3. Struggle to adapt to changing circumstances.

---

[218] Scientists Observe How New Fears Can Infiltrate Old Memories, by Esther Robards-Forbes, August 28, 2024, https://cns.utexas.edu/news/research/scientists-observe-how-new-fears-can-infiltrate-old-memories

[219] Battaglia S, Di Fazio C, Mazzà M, Tamietto M, Avenanti A. Targeting Human Glucocorticoid Receptors in Fear Learning: A Multiscale Integrated Approach to Study Functional Connectivity. Int J Mol Sci. 2024 Jan 10;25(2):864. doi: 10.3390/ijms25020864. PMID: 38255937; PMCID: PMC10815285.

[220] Maaravi Y, Hameiri B and Gur T (2020) Fighting Coronavirus One Personality at a Time: Need for Structure, Trait Victimhood, and Adherence to COVID-19 Health Guidelines. Front. Psychol. 11:576450. doi: 10.3389/fpsyg.2020.576450

[221] Westhoff, M., Heshmati, S., Siepe, B. *et al.* Psychological flexibility and cognitive-affective processes in young adults' daily lives. *Sci Rep* **14**, 8182 (2024). https://doi.org/10.1038/s41598-024-58598-3

Rigidity doesn't just affect your decision-making; it also influences your emotional well-being. Rigid self-patterns are central to various psychopathologies.[222] These inflexible thought patterns can lead to the following:

- Persistent negative self-talk;
- Difficulty in regulating emotions;
- Increased vulnerability to stress and anxiety.

Rigidity affects the neuroplasticity of your brain. Chronic stress and depressive-like behaviors are associated with impairments in neuroplasticity, particularly in the medial prefrontal cortex and hippocampus.[223] These impairments can result in:

- Decreased functional connectivity in prefrontal-limbic circuits responsible for emotion regulation, cognitive control, and adaptive responsiveness. Have you ever wondered why people living in fear-dominated environments can have strangely dissolute, irresponsible lifestyle habits they can't break free from?
- Cognitive deficits, including impaired executive function and memory;
- Rigid, negative biases in attention and information processing.

Here are some strategies to train your brain to be and stay flexible:

1. **Practice Mindfulness**: Mindfulness meditation alters connectivity patterns between major brain networks associated with self-processing and cognitive functions.[224]

---

[222] Giommi F, Bauer PR, Berkovich-Ohana A, Barendregt H, Brown KW, Gallagher S, Nyklíček I, Ostafin B, Raffone A, Slagter HA, Trautwein FM, Vago DR. The (In)flexible self: Psychopathology, mindfulness, and neuroscience. Int J Clin Health Psychol. 2023 Oct-Dec;23(4):100381. doi: 10.1016/j.ijchp.2023.100381. Epub 2023 Mar 17. PMID: 36969914; PMCID: PMC10033904.

[223] Price RB, Duman R. Neuroplasticity in cognitive and psychological mechanisms of depression: an integrative model. Mol Psychiatry. 2020 Mar;25(3):530-543. doi: 10.1038/s41380-019-0615-x. Epub 2019 Dec 4. PMID: 31801966; PMCID: PMC7047599.

[224] Giommi F, Bauer PR, Berkovich-Ohana A, Barendregt H, Brown KW, Gallagher S, Nyklíček I, Ostafin B, Raffone A, Slagter HA, Trautwein FM, Vago DR. The (In)flexible self: Psychopathology, mindfulness,

2. **Challenge Negative Thoughts**: Cognitive-behavioral techniques, such as cognitive restructuring, can help identify and modify rigid thought patterns.
3. **Embrace New Experiences**: Stepping out of your comfort zone can help build cognitive flexibility and open your mind to new possibilities.
4. **Cultivate Gratitude**: Regularly practicing gratitude can shift focus from negative to positive aspects of life.
5. **Seek Social Support**: Surrounding yourself with positive people can help counteract negative thinking patterns.[225]

The speedy quantum effect of superradiance on the one hand and rigidity on the other appear to be members of two completely different, unrelated worlds. Rigidity has been associated with depressive and anxiety disorders and personality traits characterizing conditions such as schizophrenia and autism spectrum disorder,[226] while the quantum effect seeks to heal.

Here are some strategies that may help activate tryptophan networks and potentially enhance superradiance in the brain:

Tryptophan-Rich Foods: Consuming foods high in tryptophan can increase its availability to the brain. Some tryptophan-rich foods include:

- Turkey, chicken, and fish
- Eggs
- Cheese and milk
- Nuts and seeds, especially pumpkin seeds
- Soy products
- Oats and whole grains

---

and neuroscience. Int J Clin Health Psychol. 2023 Oct-Dec;23(4):100381. doi: 10.1016/j.ijchp.2023.100381. Epub 2023 Mar 17. PMID: 36969914; PMCID: PMC10033904.

[225] Stuck on Negative Thinking, https://care-clinics.com/stuck-on-negative-thinking/

[226] Hohl K and Dolcos S (2024) Measuring cognitive flexibility: A brief review of neuropsychological, self-report, and neuroscientific approaches. Front. Hum. Neurosci. 18:1331960. doi: 10.3389/fnhum.2024.1331960

Balanced Carbohydrate Intake: Consuming carbohydrates alongside tryptophan-rich foods can enhance tryptophan's ability to cross the blood-brain barrier

Aerobic Exercise: Regular aerobic exercise increases tryptophan levels and serotonin synthesis in the brain.[227] Aim for at least 150 minutes of moderate-intensity aerobic activity per week.

Yoga and Stretching: Practices like yoga may help modulate tryptophan metabolism and potentially enhance its effects on brain function.

Consistent Sleep Schedule: Maintaining a regular sleep schedule can help regulate tryptophan metabolism and serotonin production.

Light Exposure: Getting adequate sunlight exposure during the day and limiting blue light exposure in the evening can help optimize tryptophan conversion to melatonin, improving sleep quality.[228]

Meditation and Mindfulness: Regular meditation may help modulate tryptophan metabolism and potentially enhance superradiance effects in the brain.

Deep Breathing Exercises: Controlled breathing techniques can help reduce stress and may positively influence tryptophan pathways.[229]

---

[227] Tryptophan overloading activates brain regions involved with cognition, mood and anxiety, Luana C.A. Silva , Miena B. Viana, José S. Andrade, Melyssa A. Souza, Isabel C. Céspedes and Vânia d'Almeida, Anais da Academia Brasileira de Ciências (2017) 89(1): 273-283 (Annals of the Brazilian Academy of Sciences) Printed version ISSN 0001-3765 / Online version ISSN 1678-2690 http://dx.doi.org/10.1590/0001-3765201720160177 www.scielo.br/aabc

[228] Jenkins TA, Nguyen JC, Polglaze KE, Bertrand PP. Influence of Tryptophan and Serotonin on Mood and Cognition with a Possible Role of the Gut-Brain Axis. Nutrients. 2016 Jan 20;8(1):56. doi: 10.3390/nu8010056. PMID: 26805875; PMCID: PMC4728667.

[229] Hameroff S. Consciousness, Cognition and the Neuronal Cytoskeleton - A New Paradigm Needed in Neuroscience. Front Mol Neurosci. 2022 Jun 16;15:869935. doi: 10.3389/fnmol.2022.869935. PMID: 35782391; PMCID: PMC9245524.

Complex Problem Solving: Engaging in challenging cognitive tasks may help stimulate tryptophan networks in the brain.

Learning New Skills: Acquiring new skills or languages can promote neuroplasticity and potentially enhance tryptophan-related brain functions.[230]

Near-Infrared Light Therapy: Exposure to specific wavelengths of near-infrared light may stimulate mitochondrial function and enhance superradiance in neuronal networks.[231]

Positive Social Engagement: Social interactions, especially those involving physical touch and emotional bonding, can influence tryptophan metabolism and serotonin production.

5-HTP: A precursor to serotonin, 5-HTP supplements may help increase tryptophan availability in the brain.[232]

Probiotics: Certain probiotic strains may influence the gut-brain axis and potentially modulate tryptophan metabolism.[233]

---

[230] Id.

[231] Quantum fiber optics in the brain enhance processing, may protect against degenerative diseases, April 29, 2024, https://www.eurekalert.org/news-releases/1042789

[232] Tryptophan overloading activates brain regions involved with cognition, mood and anxiety, Luana C.A. Silva , Miena B. Viana, José S. Andrade, Melyssa A. Souza, Isabel C. Céspedes and Vânia d'Almeida, Anais da Academia Brasileira de Ciências (2017) 89(1): 273-283 (Annals of the Brazilian Academy of Sciences) Printed version ISSN 0001-3765 / Online version ISSN 1678-2690 http://dx.doi.org/10.1590/0001-3765201720160177 www.scielo.br/aabc

[233] Jenkins TA, Nguyen JC, Polglaze KE, Bertrand PP. Influence of Tryptophan and Serotonin on Mood and Cognition with a Possible Role of the Gut-Brain Axis. Nutrients. 2016 Jan 20;8(1):56. doi: 10.3390/nu8010056. PMID: 26805875; PMCID: PMC4728667.

Revisit The Sleep Exercises in This Chapter

Exercise: Aligning Unconscious Goal Pursuit With Conscious Intentions

1. Awareness of Unconscious Influences

Write down three situations where you've made decisions or taken actions that seemed automatic or out of character. Reflect on why you may have made these decisions or taken these actions. Try to determine what guided you in the moment.

2. Identifying Conflicting Goals

List two long-term conscious goals you have. Then, describe any recurring behaviors or thoughts you might be taking that prevent you from achieving these goals.

3. Environmental Cues and Goal Pursuit

Examine your immediate environment (home, workplace, digital spaces). Identify and list five objects or stimuli that might be triggering goal-related behaviors, either positive or negative.

4. Visualizing Positive Outcomes

Close your eyes and vividly imagine achieving one of your conscious goals. Pay attention to the emotions and sensations this visualization evokes. Write down three specific, positive feelings associated with this imagined success.

5. Reframing Unconscious Triggers

Find one behavior that doesn't align with your conscious goals. Design a small, achievable step that could redirect this behavior towards a more beneficial outcome. Create a simple visual or verbal cue to remind yourself of this new action.

YOU STRUGGLE

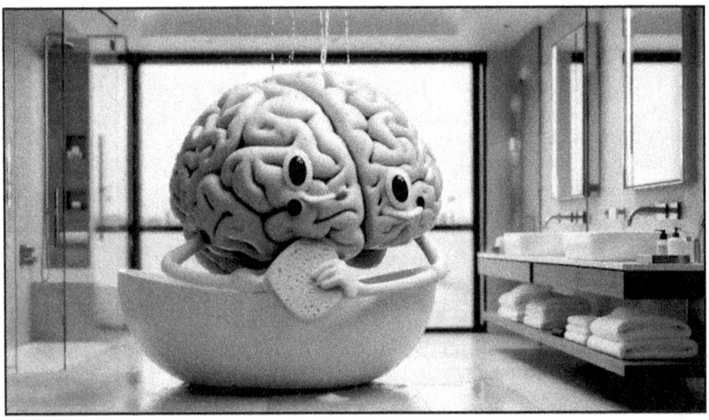

In today's fast-paced world, the adage "change before you are forced to change" has never been more relevant. That shouldn't surprise you; it's our human condition and not restricted to today's world. If you don't change your reactive thoughts and actions in the enchanted forest, the rustling in the leaves will force you to change without fail. Living a screaming life rattled by stress and fear 24/7 isn't viable for anyone. But you'll likely not experience this change you are forced to make as something you deserve. Conversely, proactive change is crucial for authentic success and how your brain adapts to new situations. Cognitive control, a key aspect of your brain's executive functions, is vital to your ability to adapt and thrive in changing environments. Recent studies have shed light on two distinct cognitive control mechanisms: proactive and reactive.

Proactive Control allows you to maintain task-relevant goals in advance of the stimuli requiring a response. It's like preparing for a storm before it hits, and you must scramble. Reactive Control is a more immediate, stimulus-driven process that kicks in when you need to respond to an unexpected event. While both mechanisms are essential, proactive control, your ability to anticipate and prepare for change, is generally more efficacious and associated with better performance in various cognitive skills.

Proactive change extends to personality traits. Individuals with proactive personalities tend to have greater career success. They are more likely to engage in development activities that enhance their abilities, exhibit higher motivation levels, and seek opportunities to achieve adequate performance.[234] In the words of Charles Darwin, "It is not the strongest of the species that survives, nor the most intelligent. It is the one most adaptable to change."

In today's rapidly changing world, the ability to not just survive but thrive during challenging times is more crucial than ever. That can be easier said than done since humans can appear wired for the negativity that stops our growth. Our brains interpret social and emotional threats with the same intensity as physical dangers. This means that job loss or relationship difficulties can trigger the same stress responses as encountering a wild animal. Interestingly, negative experiences tend to impact our brains more than positive ones.[235]

---

[234] Zhang Z, Fang H, Luan Y, Chen Q and Peng J (2022) A meta-analysis of proactive personality and career success: The mediating effects of task performance and organizational citizenship behavior. *Front. Psychol.* 13:979412. doi: 10.3389/fpsyg.2022.979412

[235] Embracing Change: The Neuroscience Behind Thriving in 2024 Insights from Grant Upbeat Bosnick (Chapter 12), https://www.achieveit360.com/embracing-change-the-neuroscience-behind-thriving-in-2024-insights-from-grant-upbeat-bosnick-chapter-12/

This negativity bias can make it challenging to maintain a positive outlook during tough times. However, understanding this tendency allows you to counteract it consciously.

Have you ever wondered about the moment you decided to make a significant change in your life? That instant when you choose to step up and start a new chapter? This process might be more complex and unconscious than we previously thought.

When you form a belief, you decide to accept a particular idea or perspective as accurate. Intriguingly, many of your decisions may be made unconsciously, including those you consider conscious choices. According to this perspective, your brain makes decisions without your awareness, and you only become conscious of these choices about half a second later. This delay between the unconscious decision and your conscious awareness of it has significant implications for understanding your decision-making processes, especially regarding major life changes.

So, if your decisions are made unconsciously, what role does consciousness play? Consciousness might function more as a memory system than a direct decision-making mechanism.[236] In other words, you don't perceive the world or make decisions directly. Instead, you do these things unconsciously and then remember doing them consciously. This theory helps explain why activities requiring split-second reflexes, like playing sports or music, seem to bypass your conscious thought processes - your conscious mind isn't in direct control of these processes.

Conscious processing plays a role, particularly in novel situations or when solving complex problems.[237] You have a sudden insight or an "aha!" moment. You experience significant improvements in problem-

[236] New theory suggests that decisions are made unconsciously, then about half a second later become conscious." ScienceDaily. ScienceDaily, 3 October 2022. www.sciencedaily.com/releases/2022/10/221003110248.htm

[237] Insights into conscious cognitive information processing, Dere Ekrem, Frontiers in Behavioral Neuroscience, VOLUME 18, YEAR 2024, https://www.frontiersin.org/journals/behavioral-neuroscience/articles/10.3389/fnbeh.2024.1443161

solving. Your mental representations are reorganized, which can also derive from unconscious memories that influence your planning and reasoning.

You may not be consciously aware of the exact moment you decide to start a new chapter in your life, but you can create the conditions that make positive decisions more likely. Exposing yourself to new experiences, cultivating self-awareness, and practicing mindfulness can influence your unconscious decision-making processes. Additionally, recognizing that your conscious mind might not be in direct control can help you be more patient and compassionate with yourself as you work towards your goals. The next time you find yourself at the threshold of a new chapter, remember that your brain might be a step ahead of your conscious awareness – and that's perfectly normal!

Have you ever felt that nagging feeling in your chest when faced with a tough decision? That uncomfortable sensation might be your heart trying to guide you toward a better future. Your heart plays a crucial role in decision-making, even if it doesn't always feel comfortable in the moment. Specific neurons in your brain's decision-making centers are dedicated to monitoring your internal bodily states, including your heart rate. This connection goes both ways. Your brain keeps tabs on your heart, and your heart rate can influence how you make decisions. When your heart races, it can alter your brain's decision-making circuits.[238]

You might be thinking, "If my heart is racing and I feel uncomfortable, shouldn't I avoid that decision?" Not necessarily! Here's where it gets really interesting. When you are faced with a decision that aligns with your long-term growth and best interests, it often triggers a state of heightened arousal. Your heart rate increases, and you might feel

[238] Study Shows How a Racing Heart May Alter Decision-Making Brain Circuits, https://www.mountsinai.org/about/newsroom/2021/study-shows-how-a-racing-heart-may-alter-decision-making-brain-circuits

a sense of anxiety or discomfort. Your body signals that you're about to do something meaningful and potentially challenging. Individuals with higher heart rate variability - a measure of the variation in time between heartbeats - tend to make better decisions in complex situations.[239]

Your decision-making process is more nuanced than you might think. Your brain doesn't make all-or-nothing choices but engages in a graded decision process.[240] This means that even as you lean towards a particular decision, your brain still weighs the evidence and uncertainty. This gradual process allows flexibility and adaptation, which can be crucial when making important life choices.

So, what does all this mean for you? When facing a decision that feels uncomfortable but aligns with your long-term goals and values, it might be worth paying attention to that discomfort rather than avoiding it. Here are a few tips to help you tap into your heart's wisdom:

1. Practice mindfulness to become more aware of your bodily sensations during decision-making.
2. Give yourself time to process important decisions, allowing your brain and heart to work through the graded decision process.
3. Remember that discomfort doesn't always mean danger - it can signify growth and positive change.

While it's true that heart-guided, growth-based decisions might not feel comfortable in the short term, they could very well have your best future interests at heart. So next time you feel that flutter in your chest when contemplating a big decision, take a deep breath and consider that your heart might be trying to tell you something important about your path forward.

---

[239] Forte G, Morelli M, Casagrande M. Heart Rate Variability and Decision-Making: Autonomic Responses in Making Decisions. Brain Sci. 2021 Feb 15;11(2):243. doi: 10.3390/brainsci11020243. PMID: 33672004; PMCID: PMC7919341.

[240] Xie, T., Adamek, M., Cho, H. *et al.* Graded decisions in the human brain. *Nat Commun* **15**, 4308 (2024). https://doi.org/10.1038/s41467-024-48342-w

In times of uncertainty, our brains often shift into survival mode. This instinctive response can lead us to "play to lose" rather than thrive in challenging situations. As we have seen, our human condition is, in its entirety, uncertain. Now you see why complaining about the weather or the job market can do you no good and won't bring answers. All you do is complain about the human condition. You should instead seek to turn that into an advantage.

When faced with uncertainty, your brain undergoes significant changes in activity and connectivity. The "confident brain" typically follows a stepwise process involving sensory processing, environmental evaluation, rule recognition, and outcome prediction.[241] However, stress and uncertainty can disrupt this process.

Uncertainty activates several key brain regions:

1. The amygdala becomes more active, heightening our emotional responses.
2. The prefrontal cortex, responsible for executive functions, may show reduced activity.
3. The locus coeruleus releases noradrenaline, increasing vigilance and attention to potential threats.

These changes can lead to a shift from thoughtful, goal-directed behavior to more rigid, stimulus-response conduct.[242] You may become less flexible and more prone to falling back on habitual responses. You "play to lose" instead of tapping into your higher self.

---

[241] Goldstein Ferber S, Shoval G, Zalsman G, Mikulincer M, Weller A. Between Action and Emotional Survival During the COVID-19 era: Sensorimotor Pathways as Control Systems of Transdiagnostic Anxiety-Related Intolerance to Uncertainty. Front Psychiatry. 2021 Jul 29;12:680403. doi: 10.3389/fpsyt.2021.680403. PMID: 34393847; PMCID: PMC8358206.

[242] Luis Felipe Sarmiento, Pamela Lopes da Cunha, Sonia Tabares, Gustavo Tafet, Amauri Gouveia Jr, Decision-making under stress: A psychological and neurobiological integrative model, Brain, Behavior, & Immunity - Health, Volume 38, 2024, 100766, ISSN 2666-3546, https://doi.org/10.1016/j.bbih.2024.100766.

The alignment between your subjective experiences (how you feel) and your physiological states (measurable bodily changes) plays a crucial role in how you handle uncertainty. This "arousal coherence" helps you maintain up-to-date representations of uncertainty in dynamic environments. For example, subtle changes in your autonomic nervous system, such as variations in heart rate or pupil dilation, can reflect changes in uncertainty. Your ability to perceive and interpret these bodily signals accurately may impact how well you adapt to uncertain situations.[243]

When you decide to succumb to uncertainty instead of striving to make something out of it and take advantage of the great opportunities it can offer, you enter survival mode, and your decision-making processes can be significantly altered:

1. **Risk perception**: Chronic stress and elevated cortisol levels are associated with increased risk-taking; you cannot navigate your life appropriately. Your ability to perceive what constitutes a risk is reduced.
2. **Short-term focus**: You may prioritize immediate gains over larger future rewards.
3. **Habitual responses**: There's often a shift towards relying on well-learned habits and routines rather than engaging in more flexible thinking.[244]

It's important to emphasize that while the initial stress response may push you towards more rigid thinking, your brain can adapt. Once the immediate stressor subsides, corticosteroid actions can help normalize

---

[243] Hannah Biddell, Mark Solms, Heleen Slagter, Ruben Laukkonen, Arousal coherence, uncertainty, and well-being: an active inference account, *Neuroscience of Consciousness*, Volume 2024, Issue 1, 2024, niae011, https://doi.org/10.1093/nc/niae011

[244] Luis Felipe Sarmiento, Pamela Lopes da Cunha, Sonia Tabares, Gustavo Tafet, Amauri Gouveia Jr, Decision-making under stress: A psychological and neurobiological integrative model, Brain, Behavior, & Immunity - Health, Volume 38, 2024, 100766, ISSN 2666-3546, https://doi.org/10.1016/j.bbih.2024.100766.

emotional reactivity and enhance higher-order cognitive processes, supporting cognitive flexibility and long-term goal adjustment.[245]

Understanding these neurobiological mechanisms can help you recognize when you are slipping into survival mode and potentially "playing to lose." By being aware of your bodily responses to uncertainty and consciously engaging your prefrontal cortex, you may be able to maintain more flexible thinking even in challenging times. To be able to do so, you must work on your decision-making, planning, impulse control, working memory, emotional regulation, attention, and goal-directed behavior. The prefrontal cortex plays a crucial role in higher-order cognitive processes and personality expression, and it does much more.

The lateral prefrontal cortex acts as a unitary system for uncertainty processing. Lesions to this region disrupt the relationship between arousal and choice.[246] To engage this area, consider different options' risks and potential rewards. The dorsolateral prefrontal cortex is involved in maintaining and manipulating cognitive representations and planning future actions.[247] When facing uncertainty, consciously focusing on organizing thoughts and creating mental models of potential scenarios can activate this region. The medial prefrontal cortex has been linked to estimating error likelihood and cognitive control in uncertain situations.[248] To engage this area, actively assess the probability of different outcomes and consider potential errors in judgment. The right

---

[245] Luis Felipe Sarmiento, Pamela Lopes da Cunha, Sonia Tabares, Gustavo Tafet, Amauri Gouveia Jr, Decision-making under stress: A psychological and neurobiological integrative model, Brain, Behavior, & Immunity - Health, Volume 38, 2024, 100766, ISSN 2666-3546, https://doi.org/10.1016/j.bbih.2024.100766.

[246] FeldmanHall O, Glimcher P, Baker AL; NYU PROSPEC Collaboration; Phelps EA. The Functional Roles of the Amygdala and Prefrontal Cortex in Processing Uncertainty. J Cogn Neurosci. 2019 Nov;31(11):1742-1754. doi: 10.1162/jocn_a_01443. Epub 2019 Jul 12. PMID: 31298634; PMCID: PMC7266503.

[247] Schmidt SNL, Sehrig S, Wolber A, Rockstroh B, Mier D. Nothing to lose? Neural correlates of decision, anticipation, and feedback in the balloon analog risk task. Psychophysiology. 2024 Dec;61(12):e14660. doi: 10.1111/psyp.14660. Epub 2024 Aug 1. PMID: 39090795; PMCID: PMC11579233.

[248] Id.

dorsolateral prefrontal cortex processes secondary value differences when predicting others' unlikely choices.[249] In uncertain social situations, consciously considering alternative perspectives and unexpected outcomes can activate this region.

"What?" You may ask. "But that's too much for me to do! I have no clue what to do when I receive conflicting stimuli or pieces of information that don't fit; this is going way too far ahead." If you have been reading this book carefully, you know by now that it is the typical survival response; it shouldn't make you feel important, needy, or particularly insightful. Note that we have just described your brain's perfectly achievable, optimal operating state. It requires you to tap into your center of higher awareness to be fully conscious of who you are in the given moment and reflect on your choices instead of being overwhelmed.

The experience differs from person to person. It's by harnessing your center of higher awareness and supporting your self-awareness that you can be conscious of the impact of your choices. Remember, while your brain's initial response to uncertainty may be geared towards survival, you can adapt and thrive. With practice and awareness, you can learn to navigate uncertainty more effectively, turning your stress and fear into opportunities for growth and resilience.

Do you want to take charge of your mind instead of letting it run the show? It's time to unlock the power of enlightened self-control and transform your life! The fascinating world of self-regulation has a significant impact on your daily life. Self-control is not just a matter of willpower, and it's certainly not meant to put you into any straitjacket. A complex interplay between different brain regions allows you to guide your thoughts, feelings, and behaviors purposefully.

[249] Ma N, Harasawa N, Ueno K, Cheng K, Nakahara H. Decision-Making with Predictions of Others' Likely and Unlikely Choices in the Human Brain. J Neurosci. 2024 Sep 11;44(37):e2236232024. doi: 10.1523/JNEUROSCI.2236-23.2024. PMID: 39179384; PMCID: PMC11403098.

At the heart of self-control lies a delicate balance between two key players in your brain:

1. The prefrontal cortex: This is your brain's control center, responsible for executive functions like planning, decision-making, and impulse control.
2. Subcortical regions: These areas, including the striatum and amygdala, are involved in processing rewards and emotions.

When you successfully exercise self-control as a mindful person, your prefrontal cortex exerts top-down control over these subcortical regions, helping you resist quick rewards processing and stay focused on your goals.[250] However, when this balance tips in favor of the subcortical areas, you are more likely to give in to impulses and experience self-regulatory failure.[251]

So, how exactly are the decisions of individuals who use self-control better decisions? They reduce cognitive overload by effectively using foresight, evaluating long-term consequences, weighing pros and cons, and employing strategies like implementation intentions and goal-setting, "if-then" plans that link situational cues to goal-directed actions. You create "if-then" plans by identifying a goal and specifying when, where, and how you'll act.[252]

You must be self-aware to use self-control effectively. Heightened self-awareness is associated with a more remarkable ability to employ constructive coping mechanisms instead of reactive responses.[253] And

---

[250] Kelley NJ, Gallucci A, Riva P, Romero Lauro LJ, Schmeichel BJ. Stimulating Self-Regulation: A Review of Non-invasive Brain Stimulation Studies of Goal-Directed Behavior. Front Behav Neurosci. 2019 Jan 18;12:337. doi: 10.3389/fnbeh.2018.00337. PMID: 30713492; PMCID: PMC6345691.

[251] Heatherton TF, Wagner DD. Cognitive neuroscience of self-regulation failure. Trends Cogn Sci. 2011 Mar;15(3):132-9. doi: 10.1016/j.tics.2010.12.005. Epub 2011 Jan 26. PMID: 21273114; PMCID: PMC3062191.

[252] The Neuroscience of Self-Control Explained, by Said Hasyim, November 4th 2024, https://www.saidhasyim.com/post/peak-self-control/the-neuroscience-of-self-control-explained/

[253] The Neuroscience Behind Self-Awareness: Understanding the Brain's Role in Self-Perception, https://www.perfectequilibrium.co/insights/the-neuroscience-behind-self-awareness-understanding-the-brains-role-in-self-perception

here is a catch: Self-control and self-awareness may compete for limited cognitive resources. Engaging in self-control tasks can temporarily reduce resources available for memory encoding and other cognitive processes.[254] Mindfulness meditation, which cultivates a basic sense of self-awareness, decreases the activity in the medial prefrontal cortex;[255] you need that activity for error-likelihood estimations in uncertain situations.

That's why, in addition to self-control for long-term goals, we importantly use cognitive control to ignore distractions, employ focus, and enhance self-awareness[256] – factors that will be very important in discussing that coveted state, the flow.

There is a strong link between self-control and mental health and a negative correlation between self-control and symptoms of irritability, depression, and anxiety.[257] Improving self-control could be a valuable strategy for enhancing mental well-being. Impulsivity isn't the key to power. Individuals with high self-control are perceived as more powerful and better suited for leadership roles.[258]

The good news is that you can improve your enlightened self-control with practice. Here are some strategies to help you flex your self-control muscle:

1. Set clear goals: Define what you want to achieve and why it's essential.

---

[254] Self-Control Competes with Memory, September 23rd. 2015, https://www.psychologicalscience.org/news/motr/self-control-competes-with-memory.html
[255] Heatherton TF. Neuroscience of self and self-regulation. Annu Rev Psychol. 2011;62:363-90. doi: 10.1146/annurev.psych.121208.131616. PMID: 21126181; PMCID: PMC3056504.
[256] Self-control and cognitive control are not the same thing, by Christian Jarrett, January 22, 2018, https://www.bps.org.uk/research-digest/self-control-and-cognitive-control-are-not-same-thing
[257] He M, Zhan X, Liu C, Li L, Zhao X, Ren L, Li K, Luo X. The relationship between self-control and mental health problems among Chinese university students. Front Public Health. 2023 Oct 31;11:1224427. doi: 10.3389/fpubh.2023.1224427. PMID: 38026364; PMCID: PMC10644003.
[258] "Having self-control leads to power." ScienceDaily, 5 March 2024. www.sciencedaily.com/releases/2024/03/240305165925.htm

2. Develop metacognitive awareness of your thoughts and impulses so you don't immediately act on them.
3. Create a supportive environment: Minimize temptations and surround yourself with people who encourage your goals.
4. Celebrate small wins: Acknowledge your progress to stay motivated on your self-control journey.
5. Engage in regular physical exercise to support overall brain health and cognitive function.

Whatever you can't handle in your life will continue to show up until you develop the skills to manage it. By strengthening your self-control, you're equipping yourself with the tools to tackle life's challenges head-on. So, are you ready to take control of your mind and shape your destiny? The power is within you – it's time to harness it and create the life you've always dreamed of!

Do you feel trapped by your thoughts, unable to break free from negative patterns or unwanted mental chatter? As you know by now, you have trapped yourself, but the key to your mental liberation might be simpler than you think. Even if self-control appears to be an abstract term, you must recognize that you have a choice. Choosing to suppress unwanted thoughts can improve mental health.[259] Practicing suppressing negative thoughts about feared future events can bring about significant reductions in anxiety and intrusive thoughts in the present. Remember this: An event hasn't occurred - until it has occurred! How many times have you been too anxious or afraid to speak up or commit to your role – until you did, and you noticed that whatever you were scared of, in fact, did not exist?

Have you noticed how easier it is to continue on your path with self-control and emotional resilience after you suppress the negative thoughts generated by your anxiety and fear? You decided to be self-confident. Do you think it is much more likely that the critic you irrationally feared

[259] Improving mental health by training the suppression of unwanted thoughts, Zulkayda Mamat and Michael C. Anderson, Science Advances, 20 Sep 2023, Vol 9, Issue 38, DOI: 10.1126/sciadv.adh5292

would have shown up if, instead, you had pulled the hood over your head to guard against your fear?

So, how can you harness this newfound understanding of thought suppression? The key lies in recognizing your ability to interrupt and redirect your thoughts. You can choose how to respond when you become aware of an unwanted thought. This concept aligns with cognitive liberty, defined as "the freedom of an individual to control their own mental processes, cognition, and consciousness."[260] By exercising your cognitive liberty, you can take an active role in shaping our mental landscape.

Here are some evidence-based strategies to help you interrupt unwanted thoughts and exercise your power of choice:

1. **Mindful awareness**: Practice noticing your thoughts without judgment. This allows you to create space between yourself and your thoughts, making it easier to choose how to respond.
2. **Thought stopping**: When you notice an unwanted thought, use a mental or verbal cue (like saying "stop" to yourself) to interrupt it. Then, redirect your attention to something else.
3. **Cognitive reframing**: Challenge negative thoughts by looking for alternative perspectives or evidence that contradicts them.
4. **Engage in absorbing activities**: Participate in activities that require your full attention, leaving less mental space for unwanted thoughts.
5. **Practice self-compassion**: Be kind to yourself when unwanted thoughts arise. Remember that having these thoughts doesn't define you.

While thought suppression can be a helpful tool, striking a balance is essential. Cognitive liberty also encompasses the freedom to explore your

[260] Cognitive Liberty, https://en.wikipedia.org/wiki/Cognitive_liberty

thoughts and emotions. Sometimes, allowing yourself to process difficult thoughts and feelings with self-control can also lead to valuable insights and personal growth.

The next time you find yourself caught in a cycle of unwanted thoughts, remember you have the power of choice. You can choose to interrupt the thought, redirect your attention, or use self-control and explore the negative thought further. This simple act of choosing can be incredibly empowering and liberating. By recognizing and exercising your cognitive liberty, we can take significant steps towards improved mental health and well-being.

Do you feel torn between conflicting thoughts or emotions? That inner struggle can be exhausting, but here's some good news: You can release your inner conflicts and find peace within yourself. At the heart of your inner struggles lies a complex interplay of neural processes. Cognitive dissonance describes the discomfort you feel when you hold contradictory beliefs or values,[261] as can happen when beliefs and values don't align with your goals. This inner conflict can lead to anxiety, guilt, and frustration. You've moved away from heart-centered decisions.

Mindfulness practices can help overcome these internal struggles. You can reshape your brain's responses to conflict and stress by training your attention inward. One key aspect of mindfulness is interoception - the ability to sense your body's internal state. Tuning into your bodily sensations can be crucial in managing mood disorders like depression.[262] Focusing on internal sensations can interrupt profoundly entrenched thought patterns and give you a fresh perspective on your emotions.

---

[261] The Struggle of Cognitive Dissonance: Mind Over Matter, https://betshy.com/2024/04/06/the-struggle-of-cognitive-dissonance-mind-over-matter/

[262] Zhou H, Liu J, Wu Y, Huang Z, Wang W, Ma Y, Zhu H, Zhou Z, Wang J, Jiang C. Unveiling the interoception impairment in various major depressive disorder stages. CNS Neurosci Ther. 2024 Aug;30(8):e14923. doi: 10.1111/cns.14923. PMID: 39154365; PMCID: PMC11330652.

Interestingly, paying attention to your breath - a cornerstone of many mindfulness practices - seems to affect your brain uniquely. Attention to breath tends to deactivate areas of the cerebral cortex involved in judgment and cognitive control[263] so you can focus on identifying that fluttering feeling in your chest instead.

Empathy allows you to understand others' pain, but it can sometimes lead to emotional burnout. There is a distinction between empathy and compassion; compassion activates reward areas in the brain independently of pain regions.[264] This makes compassion a source of resilience rather than a burden. Cultivating compassion for ourselves and others can be a powerful tool in resolving inner conflicts. It allows you to approach your struggles with kindness and understanding rather than harsh self-judgment.

Here are some practical steps to release inner conflict:

1. Practice mindfulness: Regular meditation or mindfulness exercises can help you quiet the mental chatter that often fuels inner conflicts.
2. Focus on your breath: When you feel inner conflict arising, try taking a few deep breaths and focusing your attention on the sensation of breathing.
3. Cultivate self-compassion: Treat yourself with the kindness you would offer a good friend facing a difficult situation.
4. Challenge your thoughts: Remember that not all thoughts are facts. Question beliefs that contribute to your inner conflict and look for alternative perspectives.

---

[263] Mindfulness and Meditation: Inward Attention as a Tool for Mental Health, April 15, 2024, https://www.cogneurosociety.org/mindfulness-and-meditation-inward-attention-as-a-tool-for-mental-health/

[264] The brain and peace: The role of neuroscience in resolving conflicts, https://www.berlinmoot.org/articles/the-brain-and-peace

In today's fast-paced world, it's easy to find yourself stuck in survival mode, reacting to stressors and feeling overwhelmed. This can be a problem, especially since such reactions can happen unconsciously. But the good news is that you can shift from this survival mindset to a more conscious, thriving state. Let's explore additional effective strategies to make this transition.

Survival mode is your brain's natural response to perceived threats. You easily perceive threats since the human condition is one of uncertainty, and by nature, we are wired to crave the rustling in the leaves. In this state, your amygdala - the brain's emotional center - takes control, triggering the "fight, flight, or freeze" response. This can lead to heightened emotions, analysis paralysis, and feeling out of control.[265] The problem is that due to the human need to survive and evolve, it is not only very easy to slip into this state; it can happen subconsciously. You only notice when it is too late. You appear to attract stressful, unhelpful people or events into your life without knowing why. You must make the conscious shift into a thriving state and activate different neural pathways. Here's how:

Stimulate the Vagus Nerve: The Vagus Nerve plays a crucial role in regulating your stress response. Stimulating the Vagus Nerve can help you move beyond survival mode. Known therapies to stimulate the Vagus Nerve include deep breathing exercises, meditation and yoga, humming or singing, and cold water therapy. These practices can help activate your parasympathetic nervous system, promoting relaxation and emotional balance.[266]

Practice Mindfulness: Mindfulness techniques can help rewire your brain, shifting you from reactivity to responsiveness. Regular mindfulness

---

[265] Shift Your Mindset: From Surviving to Thriving, by Daphna Horowitz, April 6, 2020, https://trainingindustry.com/articles/professional-development/shift-your-mindset-from-surviving-to-thriving/

[266] CBT Tips for Overcoming Survival Mode, September 10, 2023, https://bayareacbtcenter.com/cbt-tips-for-overcoming-survival-mode/

reduces amygdala activity and increases prefrontal cortex activity, which is associated with higher-order thinking and emotional regulation.[267]

Clarify Your Values: Understanding and aligning with your core values can help activate the brain's reward centers, promoting a sense of purpose and motivation.[268] This process involves self-reflection and can help shift your focus from immediate survival to long-term fulfillment.

Engage in Physical Exercise: Exercise isn't just good for your body; it's excellent for your brain, too. Physical activity releases endorphins, which can boost mood and reduce stress.[269] It also promotes neuroplasticity, helping your brain adapt and thrive in new situations.

Cultivate Social Connection: Your brain is wired for social connection. Engaging in positive social interactions can stimulate the release of oxytocin, often called the "bonding hormone," which can counteract the effects of stress.[270]

Practice Gratitude Regularly practicing gratitude can shift your brain's focus from threats to positive aspects of your life. This practice increases activity in the medial prefrontal cortex, an area associated with learning and decision-making.[271]

Remember, shifting from survival mode to a thriving state is a process. It requires patience and consistent practice. As you implement these strategies, you rewire your brain, creating new neural pathways supporting a more balanced, fulfilling life. So, take a deep breath, connect with your values, move your body, reach out to others, and take a

---

[267] Survival Mode: From Surviving to Thriving: Overcoming Survival Mode Mentality, June 2 2024, https://www.fastercapital.com/content/Survival-Mode--From-Surviving-to-Thriving--Overcoming-Survival-Mode-Mentality.html

[268] CBT Tips for Overcoming Survival Mode, September 10, 2023, https://bayareacbtcenter.com/cbt-tips-for-overcoming-survival-mode/

[269] Survival Mode Is on the Rise. Here's How to Identify It (And How to Break It), By Jenn Sinrich, November 1, 2022, https://www.humnutrition.com/blog/how-to-get-out-of-survival-mode/

[270] Shift Your Mindset: From Surviving to Thriving, by Daphna Horowitz, April 6, 2020, https://trainingindustry.com/articles/professional-development/shift-your-mindset-from-surviving-to-thriving/

[271] Survival Mode: From Surviving to Thriving: Overcoming Survival Mode Mentality, June 2 2024, https://www.fastercapital.com/content/Survival-Mode--From-Surviving-to-Thriving--Overcoming-Survival-Mode-Mentality.html

moment to appreciate the good in your life. Your brain - and your overall well-being - will thank you for it. With time and practice, you can evolve from surviving to thriving.

Interestingly, accepting your current experience – even if unpleasant – can lead to positive change. As psychologist Carl Rogers noted, "The curious paradox is that when I accept myself just as I am, then I can change."[272] When you practice acceptance, you activate brain regions associated with cognitive control and metacognitive awareness.[273] This activation allows you to respond more flexibly to your experiences rather than getting stuck in habitual reactivity patterns.

Learning to accept the present moment isn't about resignation or passivity. Instead, it's about developing a more balanced and flexible relationship with your experiences. By cultivating mindful acceptance, you can reduce emotional suffering, improve your ability to cope with pain and create space for positive change.

Recent neuroimaging studies have shed light on how mindful acceptance affects our brains.

1. **Emotion Regulation**: Mindful acceptance down-regulates early affective brain processes, reducing activity in the amygdala (a key region for processing emotions) when exposed to negative stimuli.
2. **Pain Perception**: Practicing mindful acceptance can reduce pain by decreasing activity in brain regions associated with pain processing.[274]

---

[272] Article: The Power of Radical Acceptance: Healing Trauma through the Integration of Buddhist Meditation and Psychotherapy, by Tara Brach, July 1, 2011, https://www.tarabrach.com/trauma/

[273] Brain Network Organization During Mindful Acceptance of Emotions, Matthew Luke Dixon, Manesh Girn, Kalina Christoff, bioRxiv 2020.03.31.018697; doi: https://doi.org/10.1101/2020.03.31.018697

[274] Hedy Kober, Jason Buhle, Jochen Weber, Kevin N Ochsner, Tor D Wager, Let it be: mindful acceptance down-regulates pain and negative emotion, *Social Cognitive and Affective Neuroscience*, Volume 14, Issue 11, November 2019, Pages 1147–1158, https://doi.org/10.1093/scan/nsz104

3. **Brain Network Reorganization**: Mindfulness-based therapies improve brain functional network reconfiguration, particularly in the executive control, default mode, and salience networks.[275]

The Salience Network is a large-scale brain network primarily composed of the anterior insula and dorsal anterior cingulate cortex. It plays a crucial role in detecting and filtering salient stimuli, integrating sensory, emotional, and cognitive information, and facilitating the switch between internally directed (default mode network) and externally-directed (central executive network) cognition.[276]

Mindfulness meditation can reconfigure the Salience Network by increasing its functional connectivity with other key networks. Specifically, one month of mindfulness training enhances interconnectivity between the salience, default mode, and central executive networks.[277] This increased cross-network connectivity is associated with improved attention regulation, emotional awareness, and cognitive flexibility.[278] These neuroplastic changes suggest that mindfulness practice may optimize the brain's ability to process salient information and adaptively respond to environmental demands.[279]

Mindful acceptance expands your attentional scope to experience present-moment sensations, whether pleasant or unpleasant fully. Broadening your attention can help reduce fixation on negative aspects

---

[275] Yue, W.L., Ng, K.K., Koh, A.J. *et al.* Mindfulness-based therapy improves brain functional network reconfiguration efficiency. *Transl Psychiatry* **13**, 345 (2023). https://doi.org/10.1038/s41398-023-02642-9

[276] Rahrig, H., Vago, D.R., Passarelli, M.A. *et al.* Meta-analytic evidence that mindfulness training alters resting state default mode network connectivity. *Sci Rep* **12**, 12260 (2022). https://doi.org/10.1038/s41598-022-15195-6

[277] Bremer B, Wu Q, Mora Álvarez MG, Hölzel BK, Wilhelm M, Hell E, Tavacioglu EE, Torske A, Koch K. Mindfulness meditation increases default mode, salience, and central executive network connectivity. Sci Rep. 2022 Aug 2;12(1):13219. doi: 10.1038/s41598-022-17325-6. PMID: 35918449; PMCID: PMC9346127.

[278] Doll A, Hölzel BK, Boucard CC, Wohlschläger AM and Sorg C (2015) Mindfulness is associated with intrinsic functional connectivity between default mode and salience networks. Front. Hum. Neurosci. 9:461. doi: 10.3389/fnhum.2015.00461

[279] Rahrig, H., Vago, D.R., Passarelli, M.A. *et al.* Meta-analytic evidence that mindfulness training alters resting state default mode network connectivity. *Sci Rep* **12**, 12260 (2022). https://doi.org/10.1038/s41598-022-15195-6

of your experience. Notice your thoughts and feelings without labeling them as good or bad. Practicing awareness can help reduce cognitive and physiological reactivity to challenging situations.[280] Regular mindfulness meditation can bring your brain's functional configuration closer to a state of mindful awareness.[281]

Cultivate self-compassion and be kind to yourself as you learn to accept difficult moments. Remember that acceptance doesn't mean approval – it's about acknowledging reality as it is. Focus on what you can change. While accepting the present moment, remind yourself that you can take action to improve your circumstances.[282]

Finding the benefit of your situation can help you exhibit higher levels of mental resilience. Even a situation that is highly unfavorable to you will have an aspect that is beneficial to you. The "you" that is aware is guaranteed to find this aspect. Some parts of this book developed from my stays in emergency rooms with a chronic pain condition years ago. Those stays cost me significant losses of resources, including the time spent that was sorely needed elsewhere. I was convinced there wouldn't be a way in the world how that could ever provide me one iota of benefit. But there wouldn't have been any other place on this planet where I could have learned what I can now use when writing this book. Nowhere else besides serving on the front lines in a combat zone, that is.

As you train yourself to find the benefit in every situation, the resilience you create will help you adapt to stress, maintain psychological health, and recover quickly from setbacks.[283] The effectiveness of benefit

---

[280] Brain Network Organization During Mindful Acceptance of Emotions, Matthew Luke Dixon, Manesh Girn, Kalina Christoff, bioRxiv 2020.03.31.018697; doi: https://doi.org/10.1101/2020.03.31.018697

[281] Yue, W.L., Ng, K.K., Koh, A.J. *et al.* Mindfulness-based therapy improves brain functional network reconfiguration efficiency. *Transl Psychiatry* **13**, 345 (2023). https://doi.org/10.1038/s41398-023-02642-9

[282] Why Acceptance is Essential in Your Healing Journey, March 12, 2023, https://hopefulpanda.com/acceptance/

[283] Bekesiene S, Smaliukienė R, Vaičaitienė R, Bagdžiūnienė D, Kanapeckaitė R, Kapustian O, Nakonechnyi O. Prioritizing competencies for soldier's mental resilience: an application of integrative fuzzy-trapezoidal decision-making trial and evaluation laboratory in updating training program. Front

finding in fostering resilience can be attributed to several cognitive and emotional mechanisms:

- **Cognitive Reappraisal**: By reframing negative experiences into opportunities for growth, you can reduce the emotional impact of stressors and enhance your coping strategies.[284]
- **Positive Emotions**: Identifying benefits in adversity can lead to increased positive emotions, which broaden thought-action repertoires and build enduring personal resources.[285]

When interpreting adverse events, your brain has a fascinating way of processing information through the lens of "YOU." Recent cognitive neuroscience research has shed light on how you perceive and internalize negative experiences and how your individual traits and tendencies shape these interpretations.

One key aspect of interpreting adverse events is your negativity bias. This refers to your tendency to pay attention to, learn from, and use negative information far more than positive information.[286] Your brain is wired to respond more rapidly and prominently to adverse events than non-negative ones.

Your personality traits, particularly neuroticism, play a significant role in processing adverse events. Neuroticism is associated with a tendency to experience negative affect and impaired emotion regulation.[287] Individuals with higher levels of neuroticism may have distinctive patterns in their resting-state brain activity following exposure

---

Psychol. 2024 Feb 5;14:1239481. doi: 10.3389/fpsyg.2023.1239481. PMID: 38374929; PMCID: PMC10875136.

[284] Id.

[285] Cao F, Li J, Xin W, Yang Z, Wu D. The impact of resilience on the mental health of military personnel during the COVID-19 pandemic: coping styles and regulatory focus. Front Public Health. 2023 Aug 9;11:1240047. doi: 10.3389/fpubh.2023.1240047. PMID: 37621610; PMCID: PMC10445488.

[286] What Is Negativity Bias and How Can It Be Overcome? by Catherine Moore, Psychologist, MBA, Scientifically reviewed by Maike Neuhaus Ph.D. 30 Dec 2019 https://positivepsychology.com/3-steps-negativity-bias/

[287] Michele Deodato, Martin Seeber, Kevin Mammeri, Christoph M Michel, Patrik Vuilleumier, Combined effects of neuroticism and negative emotional context on spontaneous EEG dynamics, *Social Cognitive and Affective Neuroscience*, Volume 19, Issue 1, 2024, nsae012, https://doi.org/10.1093/scan/nsae012

to negative emotional stimuli. Your personality can influence how your brain recovers from and processes negative experiences.

But nothing is written in stone! You can adaptively update your memories of adverse events. Through cognitive reappraisal, you can focus on finding positive aspects or alternative perspectives of negative memories to reduce their emotional impact and change the meaning of past negative experiences.[288] This doesn't change how you feel about the memory in the moment – it can lead to long-lasting updates in the memory representation itself. Focusing on the positive aspects of negative memories can lead to enhanced positive emotions, changes in memory content during future recollections,[289] fewer depressive symptoms, and more positive emotionality.[290]

Exercise: Managing Subconscious Fears

1. Body Awareness

Take a moment to focus on your body. Where do you feel tension or discomfort? This could be related to subconscious fears. Write down three areas where you notice physical sensations.

2. Emotional Labeling

When you think about a situation that makes you anxious, what specific emotions arise? Try to be as precise as possible (e.g., "dread," "unease," "apprehension"). List three emotions.

3. Cognitive Reappraisal

Choose one fear-inducing situation. Now, try to reinterpret it in a less threatening way. What's an alternative perspective that makes you feel calmer?

---

[288] Speer ME, Ibrahim S, Schiller D, Delgado MR. Finding positive meaning in memories of negative events adaptively updates memory. Nat Commun. 2021 Nov 15;12(1):6601. doi: 10.1038/s41467-021-26906-4. PMID: 34782605; PMCID: PMC8593143.

[289] Speer, M.E., Ibrahim, S., Schiller, D. *et al.* Finding positive meaning in memories of negative events adaptively updates memory. *Nat Commun* **12**, 6601 (2021). https://doi.org/10.1038/s41467-021-26906-4

[290] Wang Y-X and Yin B (2023) A new understanding of the cognitive reappraisal technique: an extension based on the schema theory. *Front. Behav. Neurosci.* 17:1174585. doi: 10.3389/fnbeh.2023.1174585

4. Curiosity Cultivation

What aspect of your fear could you approach with curiosity instead of avoidance? Frame it as a question you'd like to explore.

5. Action Planning

Based on your reappraisal and curiosity question, what small, manageable step could you take to face your fear? Plan concrete actions you could take.

SPACE AND FLOW; HACKING THE CODE OF UNCERTAINTY

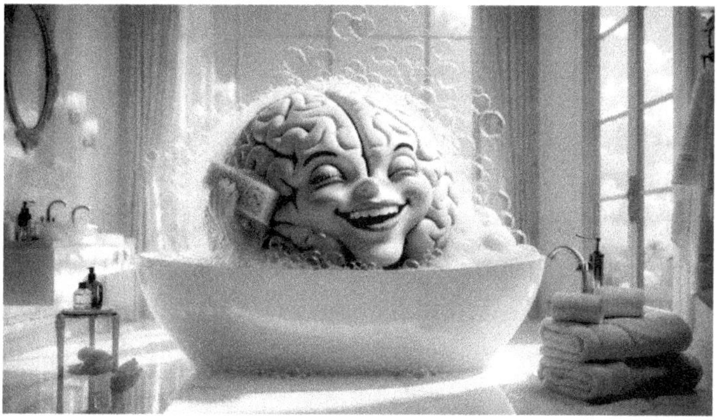

Space has an incredible reorganizing power. You have probably heard of the miraculous power of being in your own space; it can have healing qualities. You're about to find out why. Your brain creates a cognitive map to represent spatial information and help you navigate and understand your world. The entorhinal-hippocampal network makes this internal representation of space. Within this network, different types of neurons represent various aspects of your environment and your movement through it. For example, some neurons are tuned to represent your location, while others encode the speed and direction of your movements. There are even neurons that fire in response to the presence of borders and objects in your surroundings.[291]

You use spatial organization to manage cognitive control and resolve conflicts. Cognitive control is crucial for goal-directed behavior. It helps prioritize relevant information and ignore distractions. Different types of cognitive conflicts are represented as distinct points in a low-dimensional cognitive space.[292] This spatial representation allows cognitive control processes to effectively address a wide variety of conflicts by working along the dimensions of this space. Your brain uses similar spatial principles to organize and resolve various cognitive challenges.

The neural underpinnings of these spatial representations are primarily found in two key brain networks:

1. **The Dorsal Attention Network (DAN)** is involved in attentional orienting and maintaining focus. It includes regions like the medial superior parietal lobule, which activates when we shift our attention between locations or objects.
2. **The Ventral Attention Network (VAN)** interacts with the DAN when we reorient to behaviorally relevant targets; the VAN exhibits a general resetting function.[293]

Your brain's spatial information processing and perceiving and interacting with the space around you influences your cognitive abilities. Spatial cognition involves a complex network of brain regions working together. This network includes areas in the frontal and parietal lobes and

---

[291] How Do You Build a Cognitive Map? The Development of Circuits and Computations for the Representation of Space in the Brain, Flavio Donato1, Anja Xu Schwartzlose1, and Renan Augusto Viana Mendes, Vol. 46:281-299 (Volume publication date July 2023) https://doi.org/10.1146/annurev-neuro-090922-010618

[292] Id.

[293] Tosoni A, Capotosto P, Baldassarre A, Spadone S and Sestieri C (2023) Neuroimaging evidence supporting a dual-network architecture for the control of visuospatial attention in the human brain: a mini review. *Front. Hum. Neurosci.* 17:1250096. doi: 10.3389/fnhum.2023.1250096

regions like the hippocampus and parahippocampal gyrus.[294] The core network for spatial processing is symmetrically distributed across both brain hemispheres.[295] This network allows you to orient yourself in space, navigate your environment, and manipulate spatial information mentally.

Interestingly, spatial awareness is not just about knowing where things are. It's deeply intertwined with various cognitive functions:

1. **Attention**: Your ability to focus on specific locations in space involves a bilateral circuit in the parietal and frontal regions. This spatial attention helps you filter relevant information from our environment.
2. **Memory**: Both working memory and long-term memory have spatial components. The hippocampus and parahippocampal gyrus are crucial in forming and storing spatial representations.
3. **Mental Imagery**: When you imagine spatial scenes or manipulate objects in your mind, you activate bilateral networks in your brain, particularly in the parietal cortex, a brain region that plays a crucial role in attention and decision-making.[296]
4. **Navigation**: Your ability to navigate through space relies on a complex interplay of brain regions.[297] Together, these regions enable the formation and retrieval of spatial memories, allowing you to navigate familiar environments and learn new spatial layouts.[298] This spatial processing capability enhances episodic

---

[294] Spatial cognition, at https://en.wikipedia.org/wiki/Spatial_cognition

[295] Cona G, Scarpazza C. Where is the "where" in the brain? A meta-analysis of neuroimaging studies on spatial cognition. Hum Brain Mapp. 2019 Apr 15;40(6):1867-1886. doi: 10.1002/hbm.24496. Epub 2019 Jan 1. PMID: 30600568; PMCID: PMC6865398.

[296] Area of brain associated with spatial awareness and planning actions also plays crucial role in decision making, by Matt Wood, July 10th, 2019, https://www.uchicagomedicine.org/forefront/neurosciences-articles/posterior-parietal-cortex-plays-crucial-role-in-decision-making

[297] Cona G, Scarpazza C. Where is the "where" in the brain? A meta-analysis of neuroimaging studies on spatial cognition. Hum Brain Mapp. 2019 Apr 15;40(6):1867-1886. doi: 10.1002/hbm.24496. Epub 2019 Jan 1. PMID: 30600568; PMCID: PMC6865398.

[298] van Kesteren MTR, Brown TI and Wagner AD (2018) Learned Spatial Schemas and Prospective Hippocampal Activity Support Navigation After One-Shot Learning. Front. Hum. Neurosci. 12:486. doi: 10.3389/fnhum.2018.00486

memory formation and facilitates goal-directed behavior in complex environments.[299]

Your perception of space goes beyond what you can immediately see, hear, or touch. The concept of peripersonal space - the area immediately surrounding your body - and extrapersonal space - the area beyond your reach - shows that your brain represents space in multiple, action-oriented ways. Moreover, your spatial perception is not a passive process. It involves active simulation of potential actions within your environment. This embodied perception of space suggests that you enhance your overall cognitive processing by becoming more aware of the space around you.[300]

Spatial awareness plays a crucial role in facilitating higher cognitive functions and intelligence. The superior colliculus, traditionally associated with basic spatial orienting behaviors, involves complex cognitive tasks like visual categorization and decision-making.[301] This indicates that evolutionarily ancient brain structures contribute significantly to higher-order cognition. Spatial cognitive abilities have been linked to improved performance on visuo-spatial intelligence tests, which have a high loading on general fluid intelligence.[302]

---

[299] Rolls ET. Hippocampal spatial view cells for memory and navigation, and their underlying connectivity in humans. Hippocampus. 2023 May;33(5):533-572. doi: 10.1002/hipo.23467. Epub 2022 Sep 7. PMID: 36070199; PMCID: PMC10946493.

[300] Grade S, Pesenti M and Edwards MG (2015) Evidence for the embodiment of space perception: concurrent hand but not arm action moderates reachability and egocentric distance perception. *Front. Psychol.* 6:862. doi: 10.3389/fpsyg.2015.00862

[301] University of Chicago. "Activity in brain system that controls eye movements highlights importance of spatial thinking." ScienceDaily. ScienceDaily, 19 September 2024 www.sciencedaily.com/releases/2024/09/240919114439.htm

[302] The human MT complex (hMT+), involved in 3D perception processing, has been shown to play a key role in general fluid intelligence. GABAergic inhibition in hMT+ and its functional connectivity with frontal regions correlate with visuo-spatial intelligence performance. Yuan Gao, Yong-Chun Cai, Dong-Yu Liu, Juan Yu, Jue Wang, Ming Li, Bin Xu, Tengfei Wang, Gang Chen, Georg Northoff, Ruiliang Bai, Xue Mei Song (2024) GABAergic inhibition in human hMT+ predicts visuo-spatial intelligence mediated through the frontal cortex eLife 13:RP97545 https://doi.org/10.7554/eLife.97545.4

Spatial navigation, which relies on spatial awareness, engages neural networks that overlap with those involved in episodic memory and thinking about the future.[303] Spatial cognition may importantly provide a foundation for these higher cognitive functions and enhance problem-solving abilities across various domains. This integration of spatial awareness into higher cognitive processes may explain why visual representations can facilitate understanding complex information more effectively than text alone.[304]

You might tap into neural networks associated with higher cognitive functions by actively engaging with and becoming more aware of the space around you. This could enhance your problem-solving abilities, creativity, and overall cognitive flexibility.

Spatial awareness may play a crucial role in achieving a state of flow. Flow, often described as being "in the zone," is your state of optimal performance and heightened awareness. It's characterized by intense focus, a sense of effortless control, and a loss of self-consciousness. During flow, you're fully immersed in the present moment, your actions and awareness merge, and you experience profound enjoyment and fulfillment.

Flow involves specific brain network configurations and activity patterns. The hippocampus and entorhinal cortex, key spatial navigation and memory regions, support map-like spatial codes in humans.[305] These cognitive maps are not only crucial for navigation but may also contribute to the broader cognitive processes involved in flow states. The ability to

[303] Lind SE, Williams DM, Raber J, Peel A, Bowler DM. Spatial navigation impairments among intellectually high-functioning adults with autism spectrum disorder: exploring relations with theory of mind, episodic memory, and episodic future thinking. J Abnorm Psychol. 2013 Nov;122(4):1189-99. doi: 10.1037/a0034819. PMID: 24364620; PMCID: PMC3906800.

[304] University of Chicago. "Activity in brain system that controls eye movements highlights importance of spatial thinking." ScienceDaily. ScienceDaily, 19 September 2024. www.sciencedaily.com/releases/2024/09/240919114439.htm

[305] Epstein RA, Patai EZ, Julian JB, Spiers HJ. The cognitive map in humans: spatial navigation and beyond. Nat Neurosci. 2017 Oct 26;20(11):1504-1513. doi: 10.1038/nn.4656. PMID: 29073650; PMCID: PMC6028313.

mentally represent and manipulate spatial information could facilitate the seamless integration of environmental cues and task demands, a hallmark of flow experiences. Furthermore, flow states are associated with decreased activity in the default mode network (DMN), including areas like the medial prefrontal cortex and posterior cingulate cortex. This reduction in DMN activity is linked to diminished self-referential processing and mind-wandering, allowing greater focus on the task. Concurrently, there is increased activity in brain regions associated with cognitive control, such as the dorsolateral prefrontal cortex.[306]

Flow involves two key factors: extensive experience in your task, leading to a specialized brain network for generating ideas, and the release of control to allow this network to function with minimal conscious supervision. Enhanced spatial awareness may facilitate this "letting go" process, enabling you to navigate your mental landscape more efficiently.[307] To summarize, spatial awareness may contribute to achieving flow by supporting cognitive map formation, reducing self-referential processing, and enabling efficient navigation of mental representations during task performance.

When you enter a flow state, your brain undergoes some remarkable changes. One of the most intriguing aspects of flow is the decreased activity in the prefrontal cortex, particularly the dorsolateral region.[308] This area is responsible for self-monitoring and critical thinking. As it becomes less active, we experience a phenomenon called "transient hypofrontality," which contributes to the altered state of consciousness

---

[306] Tan, J., Di Bernardi Luft, C., & Bhattacharya, J. (2023). The After-Glow of Flow: Neural Correlates of Flow in Musicians. *Creativity Research Journal, 36*(3), 469–490. https://doi.org/10.1080/10400419.2023.2277042

[307] Drexel University. "Your brain in the zone: A new neuroimaging study reveals how the brain achieves a creative flow state." ScienceDaily. ScienceDaily, 4 March 2024. www.sciencedaily.com/releases/2024/03/240304135813.htm

[308] The Flow State, Mindfulness, and Mirror Neurons: Upgrading the Operating System of the Mind, by Ken Bonnet, Part I, August 2, 2024, https://kenbonett.substack.com/p/the-flow-state-mindfulness-and-mirror-neurons-upgrading-the-operating-system-of-the-mind-part-i

characteristic of flow, including distorted time perception and reduced self-awareness.[309] We act more intuitively and without overthinking. Another key player in the flow state is the Default Mode Network (DMN), which is associated with mind-wandering and self-referential thoughts. During flow, this network quiets down, contributing to the loss of self-consciousness characteristic of the experience.[310]

Flow isn't just about brain regions; it's also about neurotransmitters. When you're in flow, your brain releases a potent blend of chemicals:

- Dopamine increases, enhancing motivation, pleasure, and focus;[311]
- Norepinephrine sharpens your attention and perception;[312]
- Endorphins create a sense of euphoria and reduce pain perception;
- Anandamide, often called the "bliss molecule," promotes lateral thinking and creativity.[313]

This neurochemical cocktail contributes to the sense of enjoyment, heightened performance, and creativity you experience during flow.

At its core, flow involves intense focus and intrinsic motivation. That kind of motivation comes from within yourself, where it resonates with your identity and awareness. Flow arises through an interaction between these resulting positive emotions and high attention or focus. Intrinsic

---

[309] Gold J, Ciorciari J. A Review on the Role of the Neuroscience of Flow States in the Modern World. Behav Sci (Basel). 2020 Sep 9;10(9):137. doi: 10.3390/bs10090137. PMID: 32916878; PMCID: PMC7551835.

[310] How Are Mindfulness and Flow State Connected? https://www.mindfulnessstrategies.com/blog/how-are-mindfulness-and-flow-state-connected

[311] Id.

[312] van der Linden D, Tops M, Bakker AB. Go with the flow: A neuroscientific view on being fully engaged. Eur J Neurosci. 2021 Feb;53(4):947-963. doi: 10.1111/ejn.15014. Epub 2020 Nov 9. PMID: 33084102; PMCID: PMC7983950.

[313] The Flow State, Mindfulness, and Mirror Neurons: Upgrading the Operating System of the Mind, by Ken Bonnet, Part I, August 2, 2024, https://kenbonett.substack.com/p/the-flow-state-mindfulness-and-mirror-neurons-upgrading-the-operating-system-of-the-mind-part-i

motivation plays a crucial role in initiating and sustaining flow states. The brain's reward systems, particularly the dopaminergic pathways, are heavily involved in this process.[314]

When you are intrinsically motivated to perform a task, these systems become activated, leading to:

- Increased energy and engagement;
- Diminished feelings of fatigue or discomfort;
- A strong drive to persist in the activity.

Interestingly, the level of perceived importance you place on a task can moderate the flow experience. Flow can occur even when the challenge level is relatively low for activities considered highly important.[315] Attention acts as the lens through which flow is focused and intensified. During flow states, your concentration is absorbed in the present moment, and you are intensely engaged with your task.[316]

To build and sharpen flow states, cognitive neuroscience suggests several strategies:

1. **Find the Sweet Spot**: Aim for tasks about 4% greater than your current skill level. This creates an optimal challenge that triggers flow;
2. **Increase Novelty**: Change, unpredictability, and complexity can catch and hold attention, promoting flow;[317]

[314] van der Linden D, Tops M, Bakker AB. Go with the flow: A neuroscientific view on being fully engaged. Eur J Neurosci. 2021 Feb;53(4):947-963. doi: 10.1111/ejn.15014. Epub 2020 Nov 9. PMID: 33084102; PMCID: PMC7983950.
[315] Gold J, Ciorciari J. A Review on the Role of the Neuroscience of Flow States in the Modern World. Behav Sci (Basel). 2020 Sep 9;10(9):137. doi: 10.3390/bs10090137. PMID: 32916878; PMCID: PMC7551835.
[316] van der Linden D, Tops M, Bakker AB. Go with the flow: A neuroscientific view on being fully engaged. Eur J Neurosci. 2021 Feb;53(4):947-963. doi: 10.1111/ejn.15014. Epub 2020 Nov 9. PMID: 33084102; PMCID: PMC7983950.
[317] How to go with the flow, by Dr. Sara McKay, August 7, 2023, https://drsarahmckay.com/how-to-go-with-the-flow/

3. **Enhance Intrinsic Motivation**: Focus on tasks that align with your interests and values. This activates the brain's reward systems more effectively;[318]
4. **Embrace Autotelic Activities**: Engage in intrinsically rewarding activities – things you do for the sheer joy of doing them rather than for external rewards.[319]
5. **Set Clear Goals**: Having clear objectives for your task can help direct your attention and create the conditions for flow.[320]
6. **Minimize Distractions**: Create an environment that supports focused attention;[321]
7. **Practice Mindfulness**: Regular mindfulness practice can enhance your ability to focus attention and enter flow states more easily;
8. **Leverage Your Motives**: Flow experiences are more likely in situations that satisfy your motives, such as achievement or autonomy.[322]

Metacognition, or "thinking about thinking," is integral to the flow experience. You are aware of being in a flow state and of your beliefs about its consequences. This can influence your likelihood of entering and maintaining flow states. For example, if your beliefs about flow's usefulness for your job performance are positive, you are more likely to

---

[318] Gold J, Ciorciari J. A Review on the Role of the Neuroscience of Flow States in the Modern World. Behav Sci (Basel). 2020 Sep 9;10(9):137. doi: 10.3390/bs10090137. PMID: 32916878; PMCID: PMC7551835.

[319] The Flow State, Mindfulness, and Mirror Neurons: Upgrading the Operating System of the Mind, by Ken Bonnet, Part I, August 2, 2024, https://kenbonett.substack.com/p/the-flow-state-mindfulness-and-mirror-neurons-upgrading-the-operating-system-of-the-mind-part-i

[320] van der Linden D, Tops M, Bakker AB. Go with the flow: A neuroscientific view on being fully engaged. Eur J Neurosci. 2021 Feb;53(4):947-963. doi: 10.1111/ejn.15014. Epub 2020 Nov 9. PMID: 33084102; PMCID: PMC7983950.

[321] How to go with the flow, by Dr. Sara McKay, August 7, 2023, https://drsarahmckay.com/how-to-go-with-the-flow/

[322] Peifer C, Wolters G, Harmat L, Heutte J, Tan J, Freire T, Tavares D, Fonte C, Andersen FO, van den Hout J, Šimleša M, Pola L, Ceja L and Triberti S (2022) A Scoping Review of Flow Research. *Front. Psychol.* 13:815665. doi: 10.3389/fpsyg.2022.815665

engage in behaviors that facilitate flow experiences.[323] Remember, however, that flow involves a temporary reduction in self-reflective consciousness, allowing for deeper immersion in the task. The downregulation of explicit metacognitive processes enables more implicit, automatic cognitive processes to take over, facilitating creativity and performance. As explicit self-awareness decreases, a sense of control over the task is enhanced.

The interplay between metacognition and consciousness in flow can be understood as a dynamic process:

1. Initiation: Metacognitive awareness and control processes help initiate flow by directing attention and resources toward the task.
2. Maintenance: Once in flow, explicit metacognitive processes recede, allowing for a more immersive, less self-conscious state of awareness.
3. Regulation: Implicit metacognitive processes continue to operate, maintaining task focus and performance without disrupting the flow state.
4. Reflection: Post-flow, explicit metacognitive processes re-engage, allowing for reflection on the experience and reinforcement of positive beliefs about flow.

Flow is a state of deep focus and trust. On the other hand, self-criticism activates your brain's threat detection system and is one of the primary enemies of flow. The anterior cingulate cortex, which processes pain, error detection, and social rejection, becomes highly active when we engage in harsh self-criticism. This activation triggers a stress response.

Neuroscience offers insights into how you can break free from the self-criticism that prevents you from experiencing flow, even if you are highly experienced in a task:

---

[323] Weintraub J, Nolan KP and Sachdev AR (2023) The Cognitive Control Model of Work-related Flow. *Front. Psychol.* 14:1174152. doi: 10.3389/fpsyg.2023.1174152

1. **Cultivate Self-Compassion**: Research shows that self-compassion can deactivate the threat defense system and activate the care system in your brain.[324] This shift reduces cortisol levels and increases oxytocin, promoting a sense of calm and well-being.
2. **Embrace a Growth Mindset**: Adopting a growth mindset—the belief that abilities can be developed through effort and learning—can increase motivation and resilience. This perspective helps you view challenges as opportunities for growth rather than threats to your self-worth.
3. **Practice Mindfulness**: Mindfulness techniques can help you observe your thoughts without judgment, reducing the power of self-critical thoughts. This practice can strengthen your ability to stay present and engaged in tasks.

When you cultivate a trusting mindset, you open yourself up to numerous benefits:

- **Enhanced Creativity**: By silencing your inner critic, you create space for innovative ideas to flourish;
- **Improved Performance**: Full engagement in a task often leads to better outcomes and a sense of accomplishment;[325]
- **Reduced Stress**: Letting go of self-judgment can significantly lower your stress levels and improve overall well-being.

Developing a trusting mindset takes practice but is well worth the effort. Here are some strategies to get started:

1. **Set Clear Goals**: Having a clear objective can help you focus your attention and enter a flow state more easily;
2. **Challenge Yourself**: Choose tasks that stretch your abilities without overwhelming you. This balance is key to achieving flow;

[324] What Chronic Self-criticism Does to Your Brain, Andrea Hollingsworth, Ph.D., https://www.linkedin.com/pulse/what-chronic-self-criticism-does-your-brain-hollingsworth-ph-d-

[325] How to Master Criticism: A Neuroscience Approach to Unshakeable Self-Confidence, https://mindlabneuroscience.com/master-criticism-neuroscience-self-confidence/

3. **Minimize Distractions**: Create an environment that supports deep focus and engagement;
4. **Practice Self-Compassion**: When self-critical thoughts arise, respond with kindness and understanding.

Intrinsic motivation and attention work synergistically to create and intensify flow states. By understanding and leveraging the neuroscience behind these processes, you can more effectively cultivate flow in your daily life, enhancing performance and enjoyment in your chosen activities.

Intrinsic motivation, driven by internal rewards and enlightened personal interest, activates key brain regions associated with dopamine release.[326] This activation enhances cognitive control and attentional processes, enabling sustained task engagement. The interplay between intrinsic motivation and attention is evident in the dynamic switching between large-scale brain networks involved in salience detection, attentional control, and self-referential cognition.[327]

When intrinsically motivated, activity increases in the brain areas crucial for cognitive control and attention allocation.[328] This correlates with better performance on working memory tasks and enhanced theta band oscillations, indicating improved cognitive processing.[329] The network that supports attention, particularly sustained attention, helps create efficient attentional control and reduced mind-wandering.[330] [331]

---

[326] Ng B. The Neuroscience of Growth Mindset and Intrinsic Motivation. Brain Sci. 2018 Jan 26;8(2):20. doi: 10.3390/brainsci8020020. PMID: 29373496; PMCID: PMC5836039.

[327] Di Domenico SI, Ryan RM. The Emerging Neuroscience of Intrinsic Motivation: A New Frontier in Self-Determination Research. Front Hum Neurosci. 2017 Mar 24;11:145. doi: 10.3389/fnhum.2017.00145. PMID: 28392765; PMCID: PMC5364176.

[328] Ng B. The Neuroscience of Growth Mindset and Intrinsic Motivation. Brain Sci. 2018 Jan 26;8(2):20. doi: 10.3390/brainsci8020020. PMID: 29373496; PMCID: PMC5836039.

[329] Soliman P (2024) Unravelling the Connection between Working Memory and Intrinsic Motivation: Insights from an EEG Study. Act Psycho. 10:21.

[330] Ng B. The Neuroscience of Growth Mindset and Intrinsic Motivation. Brain Sci. 2018 Jan 26;8(2):20. doi: 10.3390/brainsci8020020. PMID: 29373496; PMCID: PMC5836039.

[331] Yun Ding, Bradley R. Postle, Freek van Ede; Neural Signatures of Competition between Voluntary and Involuntary Influences over the Focus of Attention in Visual Working Memory. *J Cogn Neurosci* 2024; 36 (5): 815–827. doi: https://doi.org/10.1162/jocn_a_02123

The resource-control theory suggests that executive control of attention toward task goals can fail over time as resources are diverted to mind-wandering.[332] However, intrinsic motivation counteracts this tendency by maintaining engagement and reducing the bias towards internal distractions. Individuals with higher intrinsic motivation exhibit more substantial and sustained theta band oscillations during tasks, indicating enhanced cognitive engagement.[333] This neural signature of motivation helps maintain focus on objectives by amplifying attentional processes and resisting cognitive fatigue, enabling you to optimize your attentional resources, leading to improved performance and sustained focus on your goals.

Keeping your mind laser-focused on your objectives can rewire your brain for success. If there is anything you have learned from the flow experience, it should be this: Give your goal your complete, undivided attention! When you set clear, specific goals, your brain responds remarkably. People who consciously set particular goals are 33% more successful than those who don't.[334] This isn't just motivational talk – it's rooted in how your brain functions.

When you precisely define your objectives, you switch on a spotlight in a dark room. This mental clarity allows you to channel focus and block out distractions that might have previously seemed overwhelming. The prefrontal cortex, responsible for planning and decision-making, becomes more active when we set specific goals.[335]

---

[332] Fortenbaugh FC, DeGutis J, Esterman M. Recent theoretical, neural, and clinical advances in sustained attention research. Ann N Y Acad Sci. 2017 May;1396(1):70-91. doi: 10.1111/nyas.13318. Epub 2017 Mar 5. PMID: 28260249; PMCID: PMC5522184.

[333] Soliman P (2024) Unravelling the Connection between Working Memory and Intrinsic Motivation: Insights from an EEG Study. Act Psycho. 10:21.

[334] The Neuroscience of Goal-Setting and Its Impact on Your Culture, September 22, 2022, https://culturepartners.com/insights/the-neuroscience-of-goal-setting-and-its-impact-on-your-culture/

[335] What Neuroscience Teaches Us About Setting Clear Goals in Performance Management? https://psicosmart.net/blogs/blog-what-neuroscience-teaches-us-about-setting-clear-goals-in-performance-management-208378

Remember, your brain can't distinguish between an authentic experience and a vividly imagined one. When you visualize your goals, you activate the same brain regions as if you were already achieving them. This mental rehearsal strengthens the neural pathways associated with your objectives, making it easier for your brain to recognize opportunities and solutions in real life. It becomes easier to stay motivated and take consistent action.[336]

You have probably heard this sentence before: "The how will show up" once you're clear on what you want. This isn't just positive thinking – it's grounded in neuroscience. When you focus clearly on your goals, you're priming your brain's reticular activating system (RAS) to notice relevant opportunities and information. Think of your RAS as a filter that decides what information from your environment deserves your attention. By consistently focusing on your goals, you're training this filter to highlight anything that could help you achieve them. It's not that new opportunities magically appear – they were likely there all along. Your focused brain is simply better equipped to recognize and seize them.[337]

So, how can you harness this neuroscientific knowledge? Here are some strategies:

1. **Set SMART goals:** Specific, Measurable, Achievable, Relevant, and Time-bound objectives provide the clarity your brain craves.
2. **Visualize success:** Spend time each day vividly imagining yourself achieving your goals. Do you crave success, but when you are asked to visualize precisely what you would like to achieve, you can't give the answer you so much thought you could give? Or do you visualize something you then feel skeptical

[336] Rewiring your brain for success: the neuroscience of goal setting, G.R. Stahl, https://www.tackletoughthings.com/blog/rewiring-your-brain-for-success-the-neuroscience-of-goal-setting#google_vignette

[337] What Neuroscience Teaches Us About Setting Clear Goals in Performance Management? https://psicosmart.net/blogs/blog-what-neuroscience-teaches-us-about-setting-clear-goals-in-performance-management-208378

or even unworthy about? Now you know why, in reality, success could be out of your reach. You must rewire your brain to give your goal the attention it deserves.

3. **Monitor progress:** Regularly track your advancement towards your objectives. This activates brain regions responsible for self-awareness and adaptability.[338]
4. **Stay persistent:** Remember that emotional regulation and persistence are key. Your brain forms connections between the prefrontal cortex and the amygdala when you set a goal that is truly meaningful for you. A meaningful goal enhances your ability to stay focused and optimistic.[339]
5. **Engage in mentally challenging activities:** Our brains don't just work harder - they work smarter. As cognitive tasks become more complex, brain activity becomes richer in detail and more streamlined.[340]

Your intuition operates mainly at an unconscious level, drawing on information you may not be aware of. You process and utilize subliminal signals to make better inferences and decisions. Without training your gut, your feelings may well lead you astray.[341] Unconscious processing is a key component of intuition, allowing you to quickly navigate complex situations without consciously analyzing every detail.

[338] Rewiring your brain for success: the neuroscience of goal setting, G.R. Stahl, https://www.tackletoughthings.com/blog/rewiring-your-brain-for-success-the-neuroscience-of-goal-setting#google_vignette

[339] Id.

[340] Fascinating neuroscience research reveals a key mechanism underlying human cognition, by Eric W. Dolan, September 19, 2024, https://www.psypost.org/fascinating-brain-imaging-research-sheds-light-on-a-fundamental-mechanism-of-human-cognition/

[341] The neuroscience of intuition and why It's Time to Hack yours, by Alexandra Jones, https://www.thestack.world/news/wellness/self/the-neuroscience-of-intuition-and-why-it-s-time-to-hack-yours-1615539839323

Several core processes contribute to intuitive cognition:

1. **Pattern Recognition**: Your brain constantly looks for patterns in your environment, which helps you make quick, intuitive decisions.
2. **Somatic Markers** are bodily sensations associated with past experiences that guide your intuitive choices.
3. **Interoception** is the ability to sense internal bodily states, which can influence your intuitive judgments.
4. **Mirror Mechanism** allows you to understand and anticipate others' actions, a crucial aspect of social intuition.[342]

By way of a side note, subconscious processing therapy, for example, uses somatic markers and interoceptions for healing purposes. If you have ever received this therapy, you most likely remember how the internal reliving of traumatic events in their altered, energy-controlled state eventually provided relief. The treatment of unconscious physiological reactivity circuits resulting from traumatic events alleviates conscious fears.[343] You may have experienced an improvement in your intuition in this process.

You can train your brain to value effort and challenge, not just outcomes. Your intuition seeks constant movement and growth. Engaging in diverse, challenging activities is one way to strengthen your intuitive abilities and keep your unconscious mind sharp.[344]

Emotions play a crucial role in intuitive processing. They act as computational tags that facilitate cognitive processes, including at an

---

[342] Sadler-Smith, Eugene, 'Core Processes of Intuition', Intuition in Business (Oxford, 2023; online edn, Oxford Academic, 23 Feb. 2023), https://doi.org/10.1093/oso/9780198871569.003.0006, accessed 2 Dec. 2024.

[343] Taschereau-Dumouchel V, Liu KY, Lau H. Unconscious Psychological Treatments for Physiological Survival Circuits. Curr Opin Behav Sci. 2018 Dec;24:62-68. doi: 10.1016/j.cobeha.2018.04.010. Epub 2018 May 4. PMID: 30480060; PMCID: PMC6251414.

[344] The Brain Loves a Challenge, Here is Why, September 29, 2022, https://www.washingtonpost.com/wellness/2022/09/29/train-brain-for-hard-things/

unconscious level.[345] This emotional component of intuition helps you make rapid decisions that benefit your well-being. Nonconscious emotional information can boost decision accuracy and speed.[346] To leverage this, you can practice tuning into your bodily sensations and emotional responses when making decisions. What does your intuition tell you, and is that how you should feel when deciding on a question? Do you experience calm alignment with your center of higher awareness? Does this help you to be a step ahead and take a view from the future?

Your brain's love for challenge and intuition's desire for movement are deeply interconnected. By seeking out new experiences and embracing challenges, you're satisfying your intuition's desires and promoting cognitive health and personal growth. Your intuition's drive reflects your brain's remarkable capacity for adaptation and development. By listening to this inner voice and continually pushing your boundaries, you're not just staying mentally fit but embracing what it means to be alive.

Intuition operates beneath your conscious awareness, drawing on a wealth of information accumulated from past experiences. For instance, researchers have demonstrated that individuals can make accurate judgments based on subliminal cues, even when unaware of them. A revealing study exposed participants to emotive images without their conscious awareness. This led them to make better predictions about the direction of moving dots on a screen based solely on these unconscious signals.[347] Your brain is wired to respond to challenges and changes in your environment. When faced with physical or psychological obstacles,

---

[345] Jellema T, Macinska ST, O'Connor RJ and Skodova T (2024) Social intuition: behavioral and neurobiological considerations. *Front. Psychol.* 15:1336363. doi: 10.3389/fpsyg.2024.1336363

[346] Intuition Training: 5 Exercises to Strengthen Intuition, by Claire Vovell, October 20, 2020, https://positivepsychology.com/intuition-training/

[347] The neuroscience of intuition and why It's Time to Hack yours, by Alexandra Jones, https://www.thestack.world/news/wellness/self/the-neuroscience-of-intuition-and-why-it-s-time-to-hack-yours-1615539839323

your intuition kicks in, allowing you to navigate complex situations effectively.

Believing is a fundamental brain function.[348] Your brain constantly integrates information from your environment with your directives, asking, "What does this mean to me?" This process forms the basis for predicting and planning your actions, including your search for purpose. A sense of purpose can act as a protective factor against various forms of suffering, including cognitive decline and depression.

Individuals with a higher sense of purpose tend to outperform their peers regarding memory and processing speed.[349] Having a purpose in life helps build your "cognitive reserve." Your brain better resists or delays neurodegeneration. Purpose doesn't just protect your cognitive abilities; it also plays a crucial role in your emotional well-being. A greater sense of purpose is associated with fewer self-reported cognitive complaints, often precursors to more serious cognitive impairments.[350]

Perhaps one of the most fascinating aspects of purpose is its ability to mediate between suffering and well-being. Meaning in life acts as a bridge between past suffering and current well-being.[351] In other words, when you can find meaning in your past struggles, it contributes to your overall sense of well-being.

Purpose also interacts with your experience of physical pain. Pain processing maintains stability through change; your mind coordinates its resources to optimize bodily functioning at different time scales.[352]

---

[348] SEITZ, Rüdiger J. Beliefs in Pain and Suffering: : A Cognitive Neuroscience Approach. *Scientia et Fides.* Online. 9 April 2024. Vol. 12, no. 1, pp. 51-71.

[349] Lewis NA and Hill PL (2021) Sense of Purpose Promotes Resilience to Cognitive Deficits Attributable to Depressive Symptoms. *Front. Psychol.* 12:698109. doi: 10.3389/fpsyg.2021.698109

[350] Sutin AR, Luchetti M, Terracciano A. The benefits of a sense of purpose in life for healthier cognitive aging. Int Psychogeriatr. 2022 Dec;34(12):1015-1017. doi: 10.1017/S1041610222000837. Epub 2022 Sep 19. PMID: 36117334; PMCID: PMC10195084.

[351] Kaftanski W, Hanson J. Suffering, authenticity, and meaning in life: Toward an integrated conceptualization of well-being. Front Psychol. 2022 Dec 6;13:1079032. doi: 10.3389/fpsyg.2022.1079032. PMID: 36562064; PMCID: PMC9763890.

[352] Philip Gerrans, Pain suffering and the self. An active allostatic inference explanation, Neuroscience of Consciousness, Volume 2024, Issue 1, 2024, niae002, https://doi.org/10.1093/nc/niae002

Individuals with higher levels of purpose in life tend to experience less pain intensity and better pain tolerance.[353]

In our fast-paced world, we often find ourselves at a crossroads where we must decide whether to take a leap of faith or wait for everything to fall perfectly into place. Embracing uncertainty and trusting your instincts can improve outcomes in many situations. That does not mean to act recklessly! Let's explore when and why it might be beneficial to trust your instincts rather than waiting for all your ducks to line up in a row.

Uncertainty is a state of limited knowledge or predictability about a situation, outcome, or future event, often involving a lack of sureness and associated with the propensity to simulate adverse outcomes.[354] Uncertainty should not appear as unusual or alarming to you, given what you know now, having read this book! Uncertainty is your human condition; you share it with every other member of the human race. You should embrace it. Your perceptions are your reality; they are the world as you see it. Your use of your cognitive processes is how you experience your perceptions. You would not want anything to be fixed, rigid, or addictively certain, given what you know now, having read this book. Uncertainty is your best friend. It is your invitation to shape your world in alignment with your authentic self. Your experience of uncertainty is a crucial cognitive skill that spurs creativity, adaptability, and resilience.[355]

"Still, my perceptions feel certain," you will say, "and I am doing this right." That's not the certainty of fixation, rigidity, or addiction. It's the

---

[353] Boring BL, Maffly-Kipp J, Mathur VA, Hicks JA. Meaning in Life and Pain: The Differential Effects of Coherence, Purpose, and Mattering on Pain Severity, Frequency, and the Development of Chronic Pain. J Pain Res. 2022 Feb 3;15:299-314. doi: 10.2147/JPR.S338691. PMID: 35140515; PMCID: PMC8820455.

[354] Anderson EC, Carleton RN, Diefenbach M, Han PKJ. The Relationship Between Uncertainty and Affect. Front Psychol. 2019 Nov 12;10:2504. doi: 10.3389/fpsyg.2019.02504. PMID: 31781003; PMCID: PMC6861361.

[355] Yearning For Certainty, November 5, 2024, https://www.beautyatwork.net/yearning-for-certainty/

moment when recognizing and monitoring your mental states and adjusting your behavior accordingly, you gain certainty in the accuracy of your decisions, memories, or predictions, and you are truly self-aware. It's the moment of ~40Hz Gamma oscillations, heightened awareness, deep focus, and sharp mental clarity immersion in your enlightened self-awareness.

It's the moment you successfully navigate uncertainty. You regulate your emotions; you are flexible; you consider the potentialities of multiple outcomes, enabling you to approach challenges creatively, adapt to changing circumstances, and build resilience.[356] [357] Your brain can perfectly integrate contextual information and episodic memory to make value-based, forward-looking decisions when outcomes are uncertain.[358] You are now on a highly improved path to make this visionary approach to the world your reality.

A war zone survivor once told me how joyful she was when she escaped the enemy. That attitude struck me as extremely strange and improbable. Wouldn't she instead tell me she crept along the ground, dived deeply into the trenches, and escaped in the night? She so wholly disagreed; she appeared not to have heard my questions. She would have done none of that; what she did joyfully meant that she was alive!

As you learn to navigate the ambiguous situation that is you, you develop the confidence to address whatever life may throw at you.[359] Your intuition processes information faster than your conscious mind. Sometimes, trusting your instincts or gut feeling can lead to better outcomes.[360]

---

[356] Surprising Link Between Creativity and Resilience, by Linda Naiman, June 13, 2023, https://www.td.org/content/atd-blog/surprising-link-between-creativity-and-resilience

[357] Yearning For Certainty, November 5, 2024, https://www.beautyatwork.net/yearning-for-certainty/

[358] Attaallah, B., Petitet, P., Zambellas, R. *et al.* The role of the human hippocampus in decision-making under uncertainty. *Nat Hum Behav* **8**, 1366–1382 (2024). https://doi.org/10.1038/s41562-024-01855-2

[359] Yearning For Certainty, November 5, 2024, https://www.beautyatwork.net/yearning-for-certainty/

[360] Drnec K, Marathe AR, Lukos JR and Metcalfe JS (2016) From Trust in Automation to Decision Neuroscience: Applying Cognitive Neuroscience Methods to Understand and Improve Interaction

Here are some more suggestions on how you can improve your decision-making under uncertainty:

- **Emotional Regulation**: The insula, a brain region involved in processing emotions, plays a crucial role in risk assessment.[361] Learning to manage your emotional responses can lead to highly improved decision-making.
- **Cognitive Flexibility**: Individuals with more significant cognitive flexibility are better equipped to address uncertain situations.[362] Engaging in activities that promote mental agility, such as learning new skills or solving puzzles, may enhance your ability to navigate risky decisions.
- **Integrative Complexity**: Developing the ability to consider multiple perspectives and integrate conflicting information improves decision-making.[363]
- **Balanced Risk-Taking**: Take the time to consider potential outcomes; your brain reflects an integration of the magnitude and probability of rewards for given risky options. This includes the probability of outcomes, the volatility of the reward environment, the variability of expected outcomes, and the engagement of cognitive control to suppress the risk-raking behaviors. [364]

Leaders and individuals alike can foster an environment that encourages taking calculated risks. Transparency and open

---

Decisions Involved in Human Automation Interaction. Front. Hum. Neurosci. 10:290. doi: 10.3389/fnhum.2016.00290

[361] Wang Y, Peng X, Hu X. Investigating the Neural Bases of Risky Decision Making Using Multi-Voxel Pattern Analysis. Brain Sci. 2022 Nov 2;12(11):1488. doi: 10.3390/brainsci12111488. PMID: 36358414; PMCID: PMC9688422.

[362] Alejandra Mitzi Castellón-Flores, Edmundo Molina-Perez Edmundo Molina-Perez, Isaac Molina, Pedro Manuel Cortes, Fernanda Sobrino, Luis Serra-Barragan Front. Psychol. Sec. Decision NeuroscienceVolume 15 - 2024 | doi: 10.3389/fpsyg.2024.1450703

[363] Id.

[364] Wang Y, Peng X, Hu X. Investigating the Neural Bases of Risky Decision Making Using Multi-Voxel Pattern Analysis. Brain Sci. 2022 Nov 2;12(11):1488. doi: 10.3390/brainsci12111488. PMID: 36358414; PMCID: PMC9688422.

communication about challenges and potential outcomes can help build trust and reduce anxiety, especially when resources and support are available for those taking risks.[365] So, foster a culture that values experimentation and learning from successes and failures.[366] Demonstrate your willingness to embrace uncertainty and learn from the outcomes. While it's natural to seek certainty and the treacherous zone of cozy comfort that comes with it, it's embracing uncertainty that is in tune with your authentic human nature. Embracing uncertainty leads to greater creativity, adaptability, and resilience.

In our fast-paced world, reacting impulsively to life's challenges is easy. However, pausing and reflecting before responding can significantly improve your emotional well-being and relationships. You can train yourself to manage your reactions effectively.

Self-regulation, the ability to control your behaviors, thoughts, and emotions, is crucial for navigating life's ups and downs.[367] It involves a delicate balance between your brain's reward centers and the prefrontal cortex, responsible for executive functions like decision-making and impulse control.[368] When you encounter situations you don't like, your brain's emotional centers, such as the amygdala, can quickly trigger a stress response, leading to impulsive behaviors if left unchecked. However, you can pause this automatic response and choose a more thoughtful reaction.[369] You may realize that the situation you didn't like wasn't what you thought it was.

---

[365] The Importance of Building Trust In Times of Uncertainty, https://whetstoneinc.ca/the-importance-of-building-trust-in-times-of-uncertainty/

[366] Good Leadership? It All Starts With Trust, by Abbey Lewis, October 26, 2022, https://www.harvardbusiness.org/good-leadership-it-all-starts-with-trust/

[367] Self-regulation for adults: Strategies for getting a handle on emotions and behavior, by Lisa Catanese, August 8, 2024 https://www.health.harvard.edu/mind-and-mood/self-regulation-for-adults-strategies-for-getting-a-handle-on-emotions-and-behavior

[368] Heatherton TF, Wagner DD. Cognitive neuroscience of self-regulation failure. Trends Cogn Sci. 2011 Mar;15(3):132-9. doi: 10.1016/j.tics.2010.12.005. Epub 2011 Jan 26. PMID: 21273114; PMCID: PMC3062191.

[369] Wang Y-X and Yin B (2023) A new understanding of the cognitive reappraisal technique: an extension based on the schema theory. *Front. Behav. Neurosci.* 17:1174585. doi: 10.3389/fnbeh.2023.1174585

Mindfulness, focusing on the present moment without judgment, is essential for improving self-regulation. Regular mindfulness practice enhances your awareness of your thoughts and emotions, allowing you to use meta-cognition to observe them without immediately reacting. Mindfulness strengthens the connection between the prefrontal cortex and the amygdala, improving your ability to regulate your emotions[370] so that your center of higher awareness can guide you.

The Stop-Breathe-Reflect-Choose approach is a practical method for training yourself to pause before reacting.[371]

1. **Stop**: When you notice strong emotions arising, pause.
2. **Breathe**: Take deep, slow breaths to activate your body's relaxation response.
3. **Reflect**: Consider the situation and possible responses.
4. **Choose**: Select a response that aligns with your values and goals.

This approach gives your prefrontal cortex time to engage and override impulsive reactions.

Improving your self-regulation skills requires consistent practice. Each time you successfully pause and choose your response, you strengthen the neural pathways associated with self-control. Over time, this can lead to more effortless and reflexive self-regulation in challenging situations. It's important to note that self-regulation may be more difficult when you're tired, stressed, or experiencing strong negative emotions.[372] During these times, it's crucial to be patient with yourself

---

[370] Marchand WR. Neural mechanisms of mindfulness and meditation: Evidence from neuroimaging studies. World J Radiol. 2014 Jul 28;6(7):471-9. doi: 10.4329/wjr.v6.i7.471. PMID: 25071887; PMCID: PMC4109098.

[371] Self-regulation for adults: Strategies for getting a handle on emotions and behavior, by Lisa Catanese, August 8, 2024, https://www.health.harvard.edu/mind-and-mood/self-regulation-for-adults-strategies-for-getting-a-handle-on-emotions-and-behavior

[372] Chester DS, Lynam DR, Milich R, Powell DK, Andersen AH, DeWall CN. How do negative emotions impair self-control? A neural model of negative urgency. Neuroimage. 2016 May 15;132:43-50. doi: 10.1016/j.neuroimage.2016.02.024. Epub 2016 Feb 15. PMID: 26892861; PMCID: PMC4851933.

and remember that self-regulation is a skill that improves as you apply and practice it.

Exercise: Setting Accurate Intentions

1. Visualize your goal:

Take a moment to clearly imagine the outcome you want to achieve. How vividly can you picture your desired result?

2. Identify your motivation:

Consider why this goal is important to you. Understanding your reasons can strengthen your commitment

3. Visualize potential obstacles:

Imagine potential challenges or roadblocks you might encounter while pursuing your intention. Mental contrasting, which involves comparing desired outcomes with current reality, can enhance goal attainment. What are 2-3 specific obstacles you might face, and how could you address each one?

4. Assess your confidence:

Rate your confidence in achieving this intention on a scale of 1-10. Metacognitive processes, including confidence, influence intention-related behaviors. If your confidence is low, what steps can you take to increase it?

5. Consider your context:

Think about the environment in which you'll be pursuing this intention. Neural representations of intentions can be context-dependent. How might your surroundings support or hinder your intention, and how can you optimize your context?

THE SUPREME CREATOR

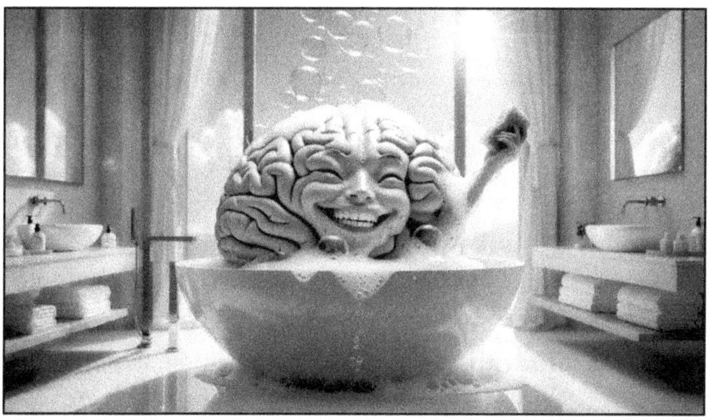

The journey of creation begins in the fascinating realm of your mind, where a simple thought, a vivid vision, or an intriguing question can spark the flame of possibility. When you focus on this new idea and commit it to memory, you set an intention - a powerful cognitive process. Intentions are more than just fleeting thoughts; they're the seeds of action planted in your brain.

When you form an intention, specific networks in your brain spring into action. The frontomedial cortex plays a crucial role in representing the content of your intentions. Two regions in this cortex blend emotion, cognition, and action seamlessly, enabling you to form, represent, and execute your goals. Mastering conflict resolution and action preparation empowers you to navigate complex decisions and turn your intentions into reality.[373] [374] [375]

You might think creative ideas come from nowhere, but neuroscience tells us there's more to the story. Slow, spontaneous fluctuations in our brain activity - the kind that happens when you're just letting your mind wander - might be the secret sauce of creativity. These spontaneous fluctuations act like an unconscious, semi-random search through all the possible ideas in your mind. When one of these fluctuations happens to land on something significant, it can cross what scientists call the "awareness threshold," leading to that "Aha!" moment we associate with creative insight.[376]

So, how can you use this knowledge to boost your creativity? Here are a few science-backed strategies:

1. **Embrace mind-wandering**: Don't feel guilty about daydreaming. Those moments when your mind is free to roam might be when your next big idea is brewing.[377]
2. **Practice mindfulness**: Regular meditation enhances connectivity in brain regions linked to creative thinking.
3. **Learn new skills**: Picking up a new hobby or language can spur neuroplasticity, opening up new pathways for creative thought.
4. **Engage in creative activities**: Regular practice in creative pursuits like writing, painting, or playing music can strengthen the neural pathways associated with creativity.

---

[373] Szekely A, Silton RL, Heller W, Miller GA, Mohanty A. Differential functional connectivity of rostral anterior cingulate cortex during emotional interference. Soc Cogn Affect Neurosci. 2017 Mar 1;12(3):476-486. doi: 10.1093/scan/nsw137. PMID: 27998997; PMCID: PMC5499751.

[374] Szekely A, Silton RL, Heller W, Miller GA, Mohanty A. Differential functional connectivity of rostral anterior cingulate cortex during emotional interference. Soc Cogn Affect Neurosci. 2017 Mar 1;12(3):476-486. doi: 10.1093/scan/nsw137. PMID: 27998997; PMCID: PMC5499751.

[375] Nachev P, Wydell H, O'neill K, Husain M, Kennard C. The role of the pre-supplementary motor area in the control of action. Neuroimage. 2007;36 Suppl 2(3-3):T155-63. doi: 10.1016/j.neuroimage.2007.03.034. Epub 2007 Mar 31. PMID: 17499162; PMCID: PMC2648723.

[376] Malach R (2024) The neuronal basis of human creativity. *Front. Hum. Neurosci.* 18:1367922. doi: 10.3389/fnhum.2024.1367922

[377] Id.

5. **Listen to frequencies**: Listening to Alpha Waves (8-13 Hz) for a relaxed, alert state of mind and Theta Waves (4-8 Hz) for deep relaxation and meditation can induce profound creativity.

Remember, creativity isn't confined to a single area of the brain. It's a complex interplay between various networks, including the cognitive control network responsible for focused attention and the default mode network (DMN) active during daydreaming.[378] This collaboration between conscious and unconscious thought processes produces our most innovative ideas.

These networks cooperate dynamically during creative processes,[379] allowing for the integration of goal-directed thinking with spontaneous idea generation, which is crucial for creative cognition.[380] In addition, functional connectivity analysis has shown increased coupling between the inferior prefrontal cortex, a key region in the cognitive control network, and core hubs of the DMN in highly creative individuals. This enhanced connectivity facilitates the generation of novel ideas by allowing for controlled manipulation of information and access to remote associations stored in memory.[381]

Furthermore, the dynamic coupling of these networks appears to be orchestrated by the salience network, which helps detect relevant stimuli and coordinate neural responses.[382] This tripartite interaction among the

---

[378] The Fascinating Link Between Neuroscience and Creativity, May 22, 2024, https://buildingbetterbrains.com.au/the-fascinating-link-between-neuroscience-and-creativity/

[379] Beaty RE, Benedek M, Wilkins RW, Jauk E, Fink A, Silvia PJ, Hodges DA, Koschutnig K, Neubauer AC. Creativity and the default network: A functional connectivity analysis of the creative brain at rest. Neuropsychologia. 2014 Nov;64:92-8. doi: 10.1016/j.neuropsychologia.2014.09.019. Epub 2014 Sep 20. PMID: 25245940; PMCID: PMC4410786.

[380] Herault, C., Ovando-Tellez, M., Lebuda, I. *et al.* Creative connections: the neural correlates of semantic relatedness are associated with creativity. *Commun Biol* 7, 810 (2024). https://doi.org/10.1038/s42003-024-06493-y

[381] Id.

[382] Kruse JA, Martin CS, Hamlin N, Slattery E, Moriarty EM, Horne LK, Ozkalp-Poincloux B, Camarda A, White SF, Oleson J, Cassotti M, Doucet GE. Changes of creative ability and underlying brain network

DMN, cognitive control network, and salience network supports complex cognitive processes, including creative thinking.[383] Flexibly engaging and disengaging these networks may be a hallmark of creative cognition, enabling individuals to alternate between focused, goal-directed thought and more spontaneous, associative thinking.[384]

Have you ever noticed how a simple question can instantly shift your thoughts? Questions have a remarkable ability to direct your focus and, in turn, shape your reality. Your brain is wired to respond to questions in a unique way. Hearing or thinking of a question triggers a mental reflex called "instinctive elaboration." This process essentially hijacks your thought patterns, forcing your mind to concentrate solely on the subject of the question.[385]

When a question is posed, it takes center stage in your cognitive processes, pushing other thoughts aside. It's as if questions have a special power to shine a spotlight on specific aspects of your mental landscape. Questions play a crucial role in directing your attention. Your ability to focus involves two key components: enhancing relevant information and filtering out distractions.[386]

Questions act as powerful tools in this process, helping you to amplify important signals while managing competing stimuli. Interestingly, this focus-directing ability of questions extends beyond the present moment. Questions can guide your attention to current sensory input, your

---

connectivity throughout the lifespan. Brain Cogn. 2023 Jun;168:105975. doi: 10.1016/j.bandc.2023.105975. Epub 2023 Apr 7. PMID: 37031635; PMCID: PMC10175225.

[383] Liu, C., Zhuang, K., Zeitlen, D.C. *et al.* Neural, genetic, and cognitive signatures of creativity. *Commun Biol* 7, 1324 (2024). https://doi.org/10.1038/s42003-024-07007-6

[384] Kaixiang Zhuang, Daniel C Zeitlen, Roger E Beaty, Deniz Vatansever, Qunlin Chen, Jiang Qiu, Diverse functional interaction driven by control-default network hubs supports creative thinking, *Cerebral Cortex*, Volume 33, Issue 23, 1 December 2023, Pages 11206–11224, https://doi.org/10.1093/cercor/bhad356

[385] Want To Know What Your Brain Does When It Hears A Question? By David Hoffeld, February 21, 2017, https://www.fastcompany.com/3068341/want-to-know-what-your-brain-does-when-it-hears-a-question

[386] Lack of focus doesn't equal lack of intelligence, By Gretchen Schrafft, Science Communications Specialist, Robert J. & Nancy D. Carney, March 8, 2024 https://www.brown.edu/news/2024-03-08/focus

memories, and anticipated future events.[387] This temporal flexibility allows questions to shape your focus across the past, present, and future.

The influence of questions goes beyond mere thought patterns - it can significantly affect your behavior and decision-making. Behavioral scientists have observed a phenomenon called the "mere measurement effect."[388] Simply asking people about their future intentions can increase the likelihood of those actions occurring. For example:

- Asking about voting intentions can boost voter turnout by 25%
- Inquiring about car purchase plans can increase buying rates by 35%
- Questions about blood donation can raise donation rates by 8.6%

These findings suggest that you can steer your actions toward desired outcomes by asking yourself the right questions.

Understanding the impact of questions on your focus and behavior opens up exciting possibilities for personal growth and achievement. By consciously crafting and asking yourself purposeful questions, you can:

1. Direct your attention to positive aspects of your life;
2. Enhance problem-solving abilities by framing challenges effectively;
3. Boost motivation by focusing on goals and aspirations;
4. Improve learning and memory by asking reflective questions.

The questions you ask play a very pivotal role in shaping your reality. When you ask the right questions, you influence your focus and reframe your perceptions in line with your intentions, influencing how you feel.

---

[387] Bringing New Focus to the Mind, December 13, 2023, https://www.cogneurosociety.org/bringing-new-focus-to-the-mind/

[388] Want To Know What Your Brain Does When It Hears A Question? By David Hoffeld, February 21, 2017, https://www.fastcompany.com/3068341/want-to-know-what-your-brain-does-when-it-hears-a-question

Asking the right questions requires willpower, especially if you are unsure about your position in the enchanted forest. People who believe willpower is self-renewing show sustained self-control, even after engaging in demanding mental tasks.[389] These individuals don't experience the typical drop in performance. It's as if their belief in an unlimited reserve of willpower becomes a self-fulfilling prophecy.

But how does this work on a neurological level? When people view willpower as a limited resource, areas of the prefrontal cortex associated with self-control show decreased activity after cognitive exertion.[390] However, those who believe in non-limited willpower maintain activation in these crucial brain regions, allowing them to continue exerting self-regulation.

Interestingly, adopting a non-limited mindset about willpower can lead to measurable changes in glucose metabolism in the brain. Glucose is the primary fuel for cognitive processes, and its efficient use is critical for sustained mental effort. Individuals with a non-limited willpower belief demonstrate more efficient glucose utilization in the brain, particularly in areas responsible for self-regulation.[391] This enables them to embrace challenges and push creative boundaries without stress and fear of depleting their mental energy.

Intrinsic motivation has a strong positive effect on creative performance.[392] When you're intrinsically motivated, you engage in activities for the sheer pleasure of doing them, which activates reward centers in your brain differently than when you're motivated by external factors.

---

[389] What you need to know about willpower: The psychological science of self-control, 2012, https://www.apa.org/topics/personality/willpower

[390] Mental fatigue leads to loss of self-control by putting brain areas to sleep, finds study, November 11, 2024, https://medicalxpress.com/news/2024-11-mental-fatigue-loss-brain-areas.html#google_vignette

[391] Audiffren M, Capa RL, Silvestrini N, Steele J, Ravel S, Pageaux B. Editorial: Effort-based decision-making and cognitive fatigue. Front Neurosci. 2023 Jun 23;17:1230022. doi: 10.3389/fnins.2023.1230022. PMID: 37425012; PMCID: PMC10327592.

[392] Fischer C, Malycha CP and Schafmann E (2019) The Influence of Intrinsic Motivation and Synergistic Extrinsic Motivators on Creativity and Innovation. *Front. Psychol.* 10:137. doi: 10.3389/fpsyg.2019.00137

The brain's mesolimbic dopamine reward circuitry is crucial in controlling reward-motivated behavior. This circuitry serves as the primary entry point for reward information. It initiates goal-directed motivated behavior by translating rewards into motivation according to their salience and is activated during difficult tasks with high rewards.[393]

Motivation is the process by which you initiate, sustain, and direct goal-oriented behavior, particularly during challenging tasks. The brain regions involved enable cognitive control to guide persistence and focus when pursuing valued outcomes.

You have discovered a powerful connection between your belief in willpower as self-renewing, harnessing intrinsic motivation, and activating states of flow and creativity. Individuals who view willpower as a non-limited resource demonstrate greater self-control and cognitive performance.[394] This mindset and intrinsic motivation can trigger a neurochemical cascade conducive to flow states by creating a sense of reward, deep focus, and pleasurable experiences linked to creative insights. You can modulate determination and self-regulation, contributing to sustained effort in challenging tasks.

This interplay between controlled and spontaneous thought processes enhances creative performance and positive emotions, broadening cognitive repertoires and creating an optimal environment for flow and creativity.[395] So cultivate a growth mindset towards willpower and engage in intrinsically rewarding activities. You can effectively tap into these neurological mechanisms for enhanced creativity and prolonged flow states.

---

[393] Weinstein AM. Reward, motivation and brain imaging in human healthy participants - A narrative review. Front Behav Neurosci. 2023 Mar 24;17:1123733. doi: 10.3389/fnbeh.2023.1123733. PMID: 37035621; PMCID: PMC10079947.

[394] Audiffren M, André N and Baumeister RF (2022) Training Willpower: Reducing Costs and Valuing Effort. *Front. Neurosci.* 16:699817. doi: 10.3389/fnins.2022.699817

[395] A psychology geek's take on creativity and how it relates to flow states, by Eva Siem, https://flowlab.com/en/mental-fitness-blog/the-psychology-of-creativity-and-flow/

You know by now that uncertainty, fear, and stress are your biggest enemies if you don't know how to play them right. The problem is that today's information-saturated media landscape thrives on the kind of experiences driving you that aren't good for you – what this media landscape doesn't want primarily is for you to be a player in it!

Your center of higher awareness is active 24/7; your authentic self watches your every thought and step, and it doesn't like what it sees. Your authentic self watches you go hopelessly astray in our contemporary media landscape. You accept novel, emotionally charged, ideologically aligned misinformation as true.[396] This creates echo chambers that reinforce false beliefs.[397] Fake news can travel six times faster than accurate news on social media platforms.[398] What is more uncertain and conducive to fear than a world that inaccurately represents what it claims is true? Your authentic self knows that the information you so ardently consume is fake.

You face unprecedented challenges navigating an environment rife with misinformation and media noise. One of the most vulnerable aspects of our cognition is our tendency to be "cognitive misers." You have two basic distinct ways of thinking and decision-making: System 1, which is automatic and requires little effort, and System 2, which is analytical and demands more mental resources. System 2 operates with self-awareness and intentional effort. System 1, on the other hand, handles the vast majority of our daily thinking processes. It relies on intuition, emotions, and unconscious processing and is responsible for tasks such as recognizing objects and faces and understanding simple sentences.[399]

---

[396] Lentoor AG. Cognitive and neural mechanisms underlying false memories: misinformation, distortion or erroneous configuration? AIMS Neurosci. 2023 Sep 7;10(3):255-268. doi: 10.3934/Neuroscience.2023020. PMID: 37841346; PMCID: PMC10567586.

[397] How and why does misinformation spread? March 1st, 2024, https://www.apa.org/topics/journalism-facts/how-why-misinformation-spreads

[398] USC study reveals the key reason why fake news spreads on social media, by Pamela Madrid, January 17th., 2023, https://today.usc.edu/usc-study-reveals-the-key-reason-why-fake-news-spreads-on-social-media/

[399] Kahneman fast and slow thinking explained, by Astrid Groenewegen, https://suebehaviouraldesign.com/kahneman-fast-slow-thinking/

You can see how your human preference for cognitive efficiency makes you susceptible to misinformation. You default to quick, easy judgments that feel right even when wrong.[400] To protect against this vulnerability, you must train to engage System 2, especially when encountering new information. This involves consciously slowing down your thought processes and applying critical analysis to the content you consume. The problem is that by nature, you employ System 2 only a fraction of the time, so you are hardly prepared. That's only the beginning of the problem.

Unexpected information tends to filter through to higher stages of processing. If you are the kind of person who likes to engage your higher-order cognitive abilities, intentionally placed, unexpected information can serve as false learning prompts. You can be provoked to accept what is fabricated to appear authentic. At the same time, when you encounter unexpected information, you tend to quiet down the expected regularities of your experiences.[401] You can fall into the pitfall of not using your abilities in those crucial moments when you need better guidance.

You are particularly vulnerable to sensationalized or outlandish claims often found in misinformation. The ability of fake news to appeal to your emotions is perhaps fake news' strongest selling point. Content spreads more virally when it contains a high degree of "moral emotion."[402] You link your emotions to your value judgments and make strong, inaccurate decisions about the information you encounter.

For example, suppose you feel strongly and positively about religion as a force that can give you safety and protection, and news with sacred connotations is presented to you. In that case, you will attach a highly

---

[400] The psychology of misinformation: Why we're vulnerable, Tommy Shane, June 30, 2020, https://firstdraftnews.org/articles/the-psychology-of-misinformation-why-were-vulnerable/

[401] Galaxy brain: The neuroscience of how fake news grabs our attention, produces false memories, and appeals to our emotions, by Rachel Anne Barr, November 21, 2019, https://www.niemanlab.org/2019/11/galaxy-brain-the-neuroscience-of-how-fake-news-grabs-our-attention-produces-false-memories-and-appeals-to-our-emotions/

[402] Id.

desirable, even sacrosanct, label to that, even if the news is fake. Moral emotion can make you highly vulnerable to manipulation. Your emotional processing systems often override your rational thinking, leading you to believe and share information that aligns with your emotional state rather than factual reality.

Are you a careful observer of misinformation? You may have noted such information can distort memories of past events and make you susceptible to false memories. [403] You may become convinced that something else happened than what you accurately thought to have occurred. And it's much more serious than that! By changing your memory, misinformation can adversely affect the intentions you set, your sense of inner space, your decision-making, and the expansiveness of your consciousness. It is no coincidence that there are no visionaries where misinformation governs! Engaging in regular physical exercise and complex cognitive tasks, such as problem-solving and strategic planning, to create a more substantial you can help counteract the effects of misinformation.

Warnings about misinformation can reduce misinformation errors. Specifically, warnings increase activity in visual regions associated with the original source of information and decrease activity in auditory regions associated with misleading information.[404] To enhance your ability to distinguish between true and false memories, you should focus on improving your source monitoring skills. This involves consciously paying attention to the context in which you encounter information and practicing techniques to attribute memories to their original sources accurately.

---

[403] Lentoor AG. Cognitive and neural mechanisms underlying false memories: misinformation, distortion or erroneous configuration? AIMS Neurosci. 2023 Sep 7;10(3):255-268. doi: 10.3934/Neuroscience.2023020. PMID: 37841346; PMCID: PMC10567586.

[404] Karanian JM, Rabb N, Wulff AN, Torrance MG, Thomas AK, Race E. Protecting memory from misinformation: Warnings modulate cortical reinstatement during memory retrieval. Proc Natl Acad Sci U S A. 2020 Sep 15;117(37):22771-22779. doi: 10.1073/pnas.2008595117. Epub 2020 Aug 31. PMID: 32868423; PMCID: PMC7502729.

Ultimately, the key to safeguarding your mind lies not only in critical thinking, emotional intelligence, and mindful information consumption. And not only with staying physically active but also with remaining vigilant about the sources and quality of the information we consume. You must do all of these. But has it ever happened that you knew the truth of information because you were an active participant when it was created at the source? Practicing techniques to attribute memories to their original sources accurately may be crucial. That factor is much neglected nowadays. You are often asked to consume information for which you can't have this accurate attribution, and that information can affect you in very profound ways.

It deserves to be noted that your ability to attribute memories to their original source accurately is not the same as having information that alleges to represent the accurate original sources, such as the name and identity of a witness that may be presented to you. Stupid creates more stupidity. If you can't be fully present with the memory, don't expect information alleged by others to be true about your memory to enlighten you!

Exercise: Nurturing Creativity Amidst Stress

1. Mindful Observation

Take a moment to observe your surroundings. Choose an ordinary object and examine it closely for 2 minutes. What new details or perspectives do you notice? How might you reimagine this object's purpose or form?

2. Temporal Distancing

Imagine yourself 5 years from now, looking back at your current stressful situation. How might your future self view this challenge differently? Write a brief letter from your future self to your present self, offering creative solutions or insights.

3. Default Mode Activation

Find a quiet space and set a timer for 10 minutes. Allow your mind to wander freely without focusing on any specific task. After the time is up, jot down any interesting ideas or connections that emerged during this period of unfocused thought.

4. Mood Shift Exploration

Recall a recent positive experience that made you feel energized or excited. How did this activating mood affect your thinking or behavior? Now, brainstorm three novel ways to approach a current challenge while maintaining that energized state of mind.

5. Cross-Domain Association

Think of a skill or knowledge area you excel in that's unrelated to your current stressor. How might principles or techniques from that domain be creatively applied to address your current challenge? List at least three unconventional connections.

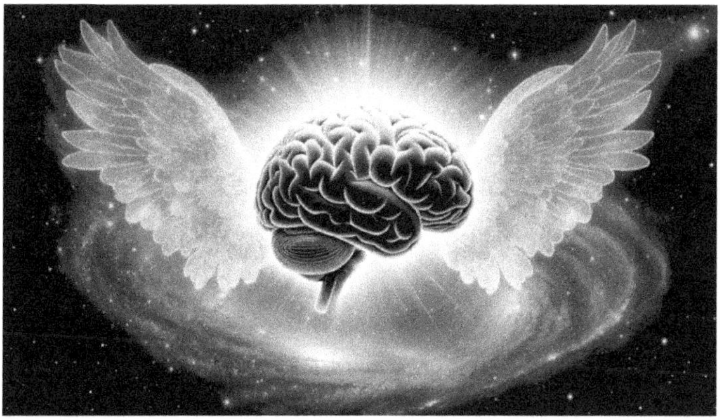

Your brain's ability to detect and respond to the many triggers of stress is a fundamental survival mechanism involving several neural nodes, including sensory, working memory, and cognitive.[405] Chronic exposure to the stress that comes with the often unconscious fears of a life built around fake environments can have significant effects on brain structure and function. Prolonged stress can rewire the brain, increasing activity in primitive parts focused on survival, such as the amygdala, while decreasing activity in areas responsible for higher-order tasks, like the prefrontal cortex.[406] This rewiring can lead to impairments in cognition, attention, and memory even without knowing it, especially when you least expect it.

---

[405] Wen, Z., Pace-Schott, E.F., Lazar, S.W. *et al.* Distributed neural representations of conditioned threat in the human brain. *Nat Commun* 15, 2231 (2024). https://doi.org/10.1038/s41467-024-46508-0

[406] Protect your brain from stress, February 15, 2025, https://www.health.harvard.edu/mind-and-mood/protect-your-brain-from-stress

Executive functions, including working memory, cognitive flexibility, and inhibitory control, are critical for navigating complex environments and deciding under pressure. These functions are primarily associated with the prefrontal cortex, an area particularly vulnerable to the effects of chronic stress.

The ability to regulate emotions is crucial in environments of perceived threats. The amygdala, which plays a central role in emotional processing, can become hyperactive under chronic stress conditions. Emotional regulation skills are required to modulate this response and reduce the negative impact of perceived threats on cognitive function.

The hippocampus, essential for memory formation and learning, is particularly susceptible to the effects of chronic stress. Protecting and enhancing hippocampal function is vital for maintaining cognitive resilience in threatening environments. Strategies that promote neurogenesis, the formation of new neurons, and synaptic plasticity or strengthening the connections and communications between neurons in the hippocampus can help safeguard these critical cognitive abilities.

Cognitive neuroscience provides excruciating detail on maintaining attention and focus in high-threat environments. Brain studies mention tonic alertness, monitoring task performance,[407] [408] sustaining vigilance, and maintaining error detection.[409] Involved are abilities of rapid response, working memory, and cognitive flexibility;[410] initiating and

---

[407] Wood JL, Nee DE. Cingulo-Opercular Subnetworks Motivate Frontoparietal Subnetworks during Distinct Cognitive Control Demands. J Neurosci. 2023 Feb 15;43(7):1225-1237. doi: 10.1523/JNEUROSCI.1314-22.2022. Epub 2023 Jan 6. PMID: 36609452; PMCID: PMC9962782.

[408] Sepideh Sadaghiani, Mark D'Esposito, Functional Characterization of the Cingulo-Opercular Network in the Maintenance of Tonic Alertness, Cerebral Cortex, Volume 25, Issue 9, September 2015, Pages 2763–2773, https://doi.org/10.1093/cercor/bhu072

[409] Farah R, Horowitz-Kraus T. Increased Functional Connectivity Within and Between Cognitive-Control Networks from Early Infancy to Nine Years During Story Listening. Brain Connect. 2019 Apr;9(3):285-295. doi: 10.1089/brain.2018.0625. Epub 2019 Mar 23. Erratum in: Brain Connect. 2022 Mar;12(2):206. doi: 10.1089/brain.2018.0625.correx. PMID: 30777454; PMCID: PMC6479241.

[410] Id.

adjusting attention; controlling spatial orienting and emotional regulation processes;[411] as well as adaptive responses and future-oriented control and present-oriented control.[412] [413]

But the minutiae of our human essence can't disguise the basics: Nature's probably oldest and most sophisticated threat detection mechanisms inside us humans. Its scientific term is the purinergic signaling system. In the intricate dance between threat perception and cellular defense, purinergic signaling emerges as an ancient, sophisticated danger detection and response system.

This evolutionary conserved mechanism serves as one of our most fundamental protective pathways. ATP, the molecule that stores and transfers energy in cells to help muscles contract, is familiar to those interested in physical exercise; it acts as a primordial "danger signal" when released into the extracellular environment during stress, injury, or threat.[414] This system is so deeply rooted in evolution that it functions as one of the most fundamental threat detection mechanisms across all cell types.[415]

Yoga emerges as pivotal for cellular harmony amidst the cacophony of modern stressors. It's also the most easily accessible; your body is all you need. This ancient practice helps your cells modulate the signals of

---

[411] Ely SL, Zundel CG, Gowatch LC, Evanski JM, Bhogal A, Carpenter C, Shampine M and Marusak H (2023) Attention, attention! Posttraumatic stress disorder is associated with altered attention-related brain function. Front. Behav. Neurosci. 17:1244685. doi: 10.3389/fnbeh.2023.1244685

[412] Wood JL, Nee DE. Cingulo-Opercular Subnetworks Motivate Frontoparietal Subnetworks during Distinct Cognitive Control Demands. J Neurosci. 2023 Feb 15;43(7):1225-1237. doi: 10.1523/JNEUROSCI.1314-22.2022. Epub 2023 Jan 6. PMID: 36609452; PMCID: PMC9962782.

[413] Cingulo-Opercular Subnetworks Motivate Frontoparietal Subnetworks during Distinct Cognitive Control Demands, Jessica L. Wood, Derek Evan Nee, Journal of Neuroscience 15 February 2023, 43 (7) 1225-1237; DOI: 10.1523/JNEUROSCI.1314-22.2022

[414] Di Virgilio F. Purinergic mechanism in the immune system: A signal of danger for dendritic cells. Purinergic Signal. 2005 Sep;1(3):205-9. doi: 10.1007/s11302-005-6312-z. Epub 2005 Jul 29. PMID: 18404505; PMCID: PMC2096539.

[415] Burnstock, G., Verkhratsky, A. Long-term (trophic) purinergic signalling: purinoceptors control cell proliferation, differentiation and death. Cell Death Dis 1, e9 (2010). https://doi.org/10.1038/cddis.2009.11

threat and danger. Yoga's transformative power extends beyond mere relaxation, reaching into the core of your stress response, soothing overactive pathways, and fostering resilience at the molecular level. Ancient science emphasizes the resultant equilibrium and a state of calm alertness that allows you to face life's challenges with grace.

As visionary leaders, we can transmute fear into resilience, chaos into order, and doubt into unwavering resolve. At the heart of this transformation lies our ability to harness the power of change, whether the brain's innate plasticity or our cell's innate drive to calmly breathe. Our remarkable capacity for change and adaptation is far more extensive than we imagine, to be found in ancient science of more than 3,000 years ago, yet in the age of machine existence quickly snuffed out.

Our minds can live in square cubicles, we have poor physical exercise, and often, we need fast results for job efficiency. Our evolutionary powers have adapted us well to living a poor quality life. Maybe for the first time in human history, our existence is encouraged to be shaped as the opposite of our authentic, visionary self. We were made to create new pathways of thought and action away from threat and toward opportunity. We should train the delicate balance between vigilance and composure to activate the seat of higher cognition, allowing for nuanced and adaptive responses instead of automated tasks.

Your true visionary's magic lies in your ability to paint a vivid picture of the future, one so compelling it ignites your brain's reward centers as a powerful antidote to the paralysis of fear. As a visionary, you understand the brain craves certainty in times of turmoil, but you also realize that turmoil is our human condition. You know to address your cravings not by false promises but by offering a clear and consistent narrative that acts as a north star, guiding your decisions and actions. This narrative, when internalized, becomes a cognitive framework that helps transform your world, using uncertainty to free up mental resources for innovation and problem-solving.

Your emphasis on long-term thinking and aligned values activates your higher-order cognitive processes. You can make the quantum leap into your state of focus and flow, where you transform immediate impulses and envision a path to success that may not be immediately apparent. Perhaps most crucially, you cultivate resilience - that vital quality that enables individuals and organizations to bend without breaking. Ultimately, the visionary's greatest achievement is weathering the storm and using it as a catalyst for transformation, galvanizing innovation, cohesion, and unprecedented growth.

Exercises: Enhancing Source Memory Attribution

1. Contextual Encoding

When learning new information, consciously associate it with specific contextual details (e.g., location, time, or sensory input). For example:

- Environment-based encoding: Study important information in distinctive locations. For example, learn about history in a museum or study biology in a garden.
- Sensory association: Link new information to unique sensory experiences. For instance, use scented candles while studying different subjects.
- Time-based encoding: Associate information with specific times of day or events. For example, review work-related material during your morning commute.

2. Theta oscillations (4-8 Hz) are involved in both memory accuracy and confidence. To implement this strategy:

During memory encoding:

- Consciously focus on generating theta rhythms in your brain by maintaining a calm, alert state.
- Visualize or imagine a gentle wave-like pattern as you process new information.

During memory retrieval:

- Take a moment to enter a relaxed yet focused mental state before attempting to recall information.
- Imagine "tuning in" to the 4-8 Hz frequency in your mind.
- Visualize the information you want to recall emerging on the crest of these mental waves.

Practice regularly:

- Engage in brief daily meditation or mindfulness exercises focused on generating and maintaining theta rhythms.

3. Sleep Consolidation

To optimize sleep patterns for enhancing source memory accuracy:

- **Consistent sleep schedule:** Go to bed and wake up at the same time every day, even on weekends, to regulate your body's internal clock.
- **Pre-sleep review:** Briefly review important information just before going to sleep to promote memory consolidation during sleep.
- **Sleep stages awareness:** Ensure you get enough deep sleep and REM sleep. Use sleep tracking apps to monitor your sleep cycles and adjust your sleep habits accordingly.

4. Emotional Regulation

Use emotional stimuli to improve source attribution for important memories stimuli:

- **Emotional tagging:** Deliberately associate important information with strong, positive emotions. For example, imagine successfully using the information in a rewarding scenario
- **Arousal control:** Practice deep breathing or progressive muscle relaxation techniques to maintain optimal arousal levels during encoding and retrieval

- **Cognitive reappraisal:** Reframe neutral information in emotionally relevant ways to enhance encoding. For instance, consider how the information might benefit your personal goals

5. Inhibitory Control

Inhibitory control plays a role in preventing false memories, especially in recall tasks. Individuals relying on intuition are more likely to create false memories. Here is how you can practice it during memory retrieval:

- Focused attention exercises: Practice mindfulness exercises that involve focusing on a single stimulus (e.g., breath or a visual object) while ignoring distractions.
- Working memory training: Engage in daily working memory tasks, such as complex span tasks, to improve overall executive function. Try solving a math problem while you remember a series of items, such as letters or words, to remember later.
- Retrieval practice: Regularly test yourself on learned information, focusing on recalling specific details while inhibiting related but irrelevant information.

"The best moments in our lives are not the passive, receptive, relaxing times . . . The best moments usually occur if a person's body or mind is stretched to its limits in a voluntary effort to accomplish something difficult and worthwhile."

(Mihaly Csikszentmihalyi, 1990)[416]

---

[416] 8 Traits of Flow According to Mihaly Csikszentmihalyi, by Mike Oppland, BA, MBA, 16 Dec 2016, https://positivepsychology.com/mihaly-csikszentmihalyi-father-of-flow/

www.ingramcontent.com/pod-product-compliance
Lightning Source LLC
LaVergne TN
LVHW022219200926
848481LV00006B/2033
* 9 7 9 8 9 9 1 8 8 6 2 4 6 *